THE BEHAVIOUR CHAIN PRINCIPLE

Understanding Why People Do What They Do

Joanne Eussen

Registered Nurse, Master of Mental Health Nursing

Founder of The Resilience Echo

For every support worker, clinician, peer worker, and carer who has ever stood in a difficult moment and wondered:

what just happened?

This book is for you.

The Behaviour Chain Principle

Understanding Why People Do What They Do

First published 2026

The Resilience Echo

www.theresilienceecho.com

ISBN 978-1-7646063-0-1 (paperback)

CONTENTS

Introduction

PART ONE

Understanding the Chain

PART TWO

Walking the Chain

PART THREE

Working with the Chain

Conclusion

Appendix

INTRODUCTION

I have spent sixteen years as a Mental Health Nurse working on the frontline in acute mental health settings. I hold a nursing degree and a Master's in Mental Health Nursing. But the idea at the centre of this book did not come from a lecture theatre or a research paper.

It came from the wards. From the moments that no training manual fully prepares you for.

I have sat with people experiencing suicidal ideation, severe emotional dysregulation, psychosis, and complex behavioural presentations. I have seen behaviour that frightened people, confused people, and broke the hearts of the people trying hardest to help.

And across all of that, one thing has stayed with me.

The people doing the most direct, most demanding work, the support workers and frontline carers who show up day after day into other people's lives, are often doing it without the tools they need to understand what they are actually dealing with.

They are given procedures, risk assessments, and support plans written in careful professional language that describes what a person needs without always explaining why they do what they do. And then they walk through a door, into a real situation, and they are expected to manage.

By the time acute mental health clinicians become involved, they are frequently managing two people. The participant in significant distress, and the support worker carrying responsibility beyond what can be safely managed. Emergency services are drawn in. Outcomes that could have been prevented were not, because the early response did not have a framework to stand on.

That is the gap this book exists to fill.

Through The Resilience Echo I have developed clinician-led training for frontline workers, disability support teams, and the organisations that employ them. That work has reinforced what I first observed in acute settings. When workers share the same framework for understanding behaviour, something changes.

Responses become steadier. Escalations reduce. Workers feel supported rather than exposed.

The Behaviour Chain Principle is that framework. It begins with a single idea.

Behaviour is never the beginning of the story.

What looks sudden from the outside has been forming, quietly and inevitably, long before anyone watching could see it. Once you understand that, everything about how you respond begins to change.

This book is for the support worker who has wondered what just happened. For the team leader trying to make sense of patterns that keep repeating. For the clinician, the peer worker, and the service provider who wants to build something better. It is built in three parts, with a practical appendix designed to be used, not filed away.

One final thing. This framework will ask you to look at your own chain, not just the chains of the people you support. It is not a comfortable invitation. But it is an honest one. The workers willing to look at their own chain are the ones who change things, for the people they support, and for themselves.

I hope this book gives you a new way of seeing behaviour.

Joanne Eussen

Registered Nurse, Master of Mental Health Nursing

Founder of The Resilience Echo

THE BEHAVIOUR CHAIN PRINCIPLE

Understanding Why People Do What They Do

CHAPTER ONE

The Behaviour Chain Principle

Have you ever been in a conversation when something that was said touched a nerve or triggered a response you were not expecting?

You reacted quickly.

You said something sharp.

You withdrew from the conversation or changed your tone.

Later, when you had time to reflect, you questioned your reaction.

Why did that affect me so strongly?

What happened in that moment between hearing those words and responding to them?

Can you remember what you felt at the time?

And if you can remember the feeling, do you know where it came from?

How did your internal experience shift from the moment you first heard the words to the moment your behaviour changed?

To the outside world, behaviour often appears suddenly.

A comment is made.

A look is exchanged.

A message is received.

And something shifts inside us.

But behaviour rarely begins where we think it does.

What we see on the surface is often only the final, and sometimes fragile, link in a much longer chain of events. A chain that has been quietly forming long before the behaviour itself appears.

This is where the Behaviour Chain Principle begins.

The Behaviour Chain Principle is neither rare nor unusual. In fact, it is something we witness every day.

Yet while the chain itself is universal, the links within it are deeply individual.

Each person carries their own interpretations, memories, expectations, and emotional experiences into every interaction. These influences shape how we understand what is happening around us and how we decide to respond.

Sometimes the chain reveals only a brief glimpse of someone's character.

At other times it reflects the weight of experiences they have carried into that moment.

Behaviour, then, is not simply a reaction.

It is the visible outcome of everything that has already taken place within the chain.

Consider a community support worker organising an outing for a client who would rather stay home gaming.

The worker encourages the idea gently at first. They offer choices and explain the benefits of getting outside, fresh air, a change of environment, an opportunity to enjoy the day.

The client refuses.

They want to stay home and continue gaming.

The worker tries again, hoping a little encouragement might help. Another suggestion is offered. Another reason to go out is explained.

But something begins to change.

The client may interpret what the worker experiences as encouragement in a completely different way. What was intended as support can feel like pressure.

Inside the client's experience, several things may already be happening.

Their expectation for the day has shifted.

Someone is challenging their preferred activity.

They may anticipate further insistence.

Each of these influences adds pressure to the chain.

The worker continues to encourage the outing, unaware that the chain is already under strain.

Then the fragile link gives way.

The client becomes dysregulated and creates a scene. The behaviour escalates quickly, and the worker decides to stop insisting in order to calm the situation.

From the outside, the behaviour can appear sudden.

But the behaviour was not the beginning of the event.

It was the end of it.

Pressure had already been building within the chain long before the behaviour appeared.

The internal experience of reaching that fragile link in the chain can feel vastly different from the way the situation appears to someone watching it unfold. The difference between living the moment and observing it can be considerable.

In some situations, the behaviour achieves the desired outcome. The worker backs away and the outing is cancelled.

When this happens repeatedly, the behaviour can become reinforced.

Over time the person learns that escalating their response changes the situation around them. What may begin as an emotional reaction can gradually become a learned strategy for influencing the outcome of future interactions.

Understanding the Behaviour Chain Principle helps us recognise these moments earlier. Instead of focusing only on the behaviour that appears at the end of the chain, we begin to see the influences that were building long before the fragile link gave way.

Watching these changes from the outside, particularly in a care-related role, can often lead to confusion and frustration.

To the observer, the behaviour may appear sudden or exaggerated. It can feel as though the person has overreacted or is deliberately creating difficulty.

Judgements can quickly follow, often expressed in comments such as:

"They overreacted."

"They're difficult."

"They're manipulative."

When situations escalate repeatedly, it can become increasingly challenging for carers or support workers to maintain engagement. Behaviour that consistently escalates to the point where the worker feels forced to step away in order to keep the peace can create ongoing strain in the relationship.

Over time, these situations may lead to reduced support, withdrawal of services, or unused care packages. When this happens, the person at the centre of the behaviour may become more vulnerable rather than more supported.

Understanding the Behaviour Chain Principle helps shift the focus away from judging the behaviour itself and toward recognising the pressures building within the chain long before the behaviour appears.

By the time a client escalates into a noticeable change in behaviour, they have already moved through multiple links in the behaviour chain.

Each of these links is shaped by the individual and the circumstances surrounding the moment. Interpretation, past experience, expectation, and emotion all influence how a situation is understood and how a response begins to form.

Recognising these links, both by the client and by those supporting them, can become a valuable tool in managing behaviour. When the early signs of pressure within the chain are noticed, adjustments can sometimes be made to the environment, the communication, or the approach being used.

Even minor changes can reduce the strain on the chain before it reaches the fragile link.

However, when additional influences are present, such as past experiences or unresolved emotional triggers, pressure can build rapidly. What might appear to be a calm situation can shift quickly, pushing the chain toward its weakest point.

When that fragile link gives way, behaviour changes.

Imagine, for a moment, a length of chain made up of many individual links.

Now imagine that every person carries their own chain. No two are identical.

Some of the links remain constant throughout life. Others change depending on circumstances, environment, and experiences.

While the chain may be influenced by external pressures or stimuli, the actions that eventually emerge from it are experienced and expressed by the person who carries it.

Within the Behaviour Chain Principle, these links can be thought of as either static or dynamic.

Static links are the aspects of a person's life that are fixed or deeply established. They shape how the person experiences the world but are not easily changed.

Examples of static links may include:

Gender.

Age.

History of trauma.

Childhood experiences.

Family dynamics.

Dynamic links, on the other hand, are influences that can shift depending on the situation, environment, or a person's current state.

Examples of dynamic links may include:

Environment.

Illness or disorders.

Medications.

Substance use.

External contacts such as supports or family.

Engagement with treatment.

Insight.

Understanding of a situation.

Capacity to make decisions.

When several of these links are active within a situation, pressure within the chain can increase rapidly.

Returning to our earlier example of the client who prefers to stay home gaming, it becomes easier to see how multiple links may already be under strain before the worker even suggests the outing.

A disrupted routine, previous experiences of being pressured, medication effects, or environmental stressors may all be influencing the chain.

When enough of these influences align, the chain moves closer to its fragile point.

And when that fragile link gives way, behaviour changes.

At times, a client may have been supported by a service that introduced clear boundaries and expectations around behaviour from the beginning. When this occurs, the behaviour chain can respond very differently.

Clear and consistent boundaries strengthen the links within the chain. Both the client and the worker understand what is expected, and this shared understanding often reduces the likelihood of escalation.

Changes in behaviour may still occur from time to time. This is part of being human. But the chain is less likely to reach the fragile point where behaviour becomes highly reactive.

When expectations are consistent and well understood by both the client and the worker, there is less opportunity for behaviour to develop into patterns that attempt to control or influence outcomes.

Small ruptures may still occur, but they tend to be occasional rather than constant. In many cases they can even be anticipated when the worker understands the Behaviour Chain Principle and recognises the pressure building within the chain.

The complexity of managing behaviour also includes the reactions, and the behaviour chains, of the person delivering the care.

Support workers are not separate from the situation. They bring their own experiences, interpretations, expectations, and emotional responses into the interaction.

Two workers may respond very differently to the same situation. One may remain calm and help settle the moment, while another may unintentionally escalate it based on their own understanding, past experiences, or emotional response at the time.

When responses vary significantly between workers, boundaries can become unclear. If the whole team is not approaching the situation in a consistent way, the client may experience mixed expectations, which can place additional strain on the behaviour chain.

In some circumstances, escalating situations may result in increased involvement from emergency services or unnecessary hospital presentations when the behaviour has reached a point where the environment can no longer manage the escalation safely.

The impact of these situations is not limited to the client. Workers themselves experience pressure within their own behaviour chains.

After difficult interactions, support workers often need time to debrief, reflect, and reset. Allowing space for this process helps the worker restore balance within their own chain before returning to care delivery.

Reflection: Noticing the Chain in Your Own Experience

Think of a recent moment when someone's behaviour surprised you.

It may have been a client, a colleague, a family member, or someone you encountered briefly.

The behaviour arrived, and your first response was to the behaviour itself.

Without analysing the situation in detail, pause and consider the following.

What do you think was happening for that person before the behaviour appeared?

What in their environment, their history, or their current state might have been shaping the moment?

And what was happening in you as you watched it unfold?

This reflection is not about finding the right answer.

It is about beginning to look earlier.

That habit of looking before the behaviour, not only at it, is what the rest of this book is built to develop.

Closing: The Chain as a Way of Seeing

The Behaviour Chain Principle begins with a single shift.

Not in technique. Not in policy. Not in procedure.

In perspective.

When behaviour is understood as the final link in a chain, not the beginning of an event, everything about how we respond begins to change.

The question stops being: why did this person behave this way?

It becomes: what were the links that led here?

That question does not excuse behaviour.

It does not remove accountability.

It opens something more useful than judgement.

It opens understanding.

The chapters ahead will walk the full length of the chain, link by link. Each one shapes the next. Each one carries the weight of everything that came before it.

By the time behaviour appears, the chain has already done most of its work.

Learning to see that work before behaviour makes it visible is where everything changes.

Behaviour rarely begins where we think it does.

By the time a reaction becomes visible, the chain has already been forming. Interpretation, memory, expectation, emotion, and circumstance have already been moving through the links.

The fragile point we eventually witness is not the beginning of the event.

It is the end of it.

Understanding this changes how we see behaviour.

Instead of focusing only on the reaction, we begin to look earlier in the chain, at the influences, pressures, and experiences that shape the moment before behaviour appears.

And once we begin to see the chain, we start to recognise something important.

Behaviour is rarely random.

It is connected.

The real question, then, is not simply why behaviour happened.

It is this.

What were the links that led to it?

CHAPTER TWO

Environment

The Setting That Shapes the Chain

To understand behaviour, we first need to see the chain that leads to it.

ENVIRONMENT → INTERPRETATION → MEMORY → UNDERSTANDING → EMOTION → EXPECTATION → BEHAVIOUR

Behaviour is the final link in the chain.

This sequence is presented as linear because that is how it is most clearly understood. In practice, these links do not always wait neatly for each other. Emotion can sharpen interpretation. Memory can colour understanding before understanding has fully formed. The chain is a tool for thinking, not a diagram of machinery. What matters is not perfect precision but the habit of looking earlier, of asking what was already moving through the chain before the behaviour appeared.

Each of these links will be explored in the chapters ahead. Together they form the full sequence through which external events become internal experiences, and internal experiences become visible behaviour.

The arrangement and influence of each link within the behaviour chain is unique to the individual. These domains of influence include both static elements, such as past experiences or long-standing beliefs, and dynamic elements, such as current environment, physical state, or situational stress.

Because these influences are fluid, the relative strength of each link can shift from moment to moment.

Emotional responses connected to these links play a significant role in how the chain functions. A person's capacity to recognise, tolerate, and regulate emotional activation can either stabilise the chain or contribute to increasing strain. When emotional regulation is reduced, the overall resilience of the chain may weaken, making behavioural change more likely to occur.

In this way, behaviour is not simply a reaction to a single moment. It is the visible expression of shifting pressures within an individual behavioural system.

Because the influence of each link is fluid and individual, behavioural strain often becomes most visible when a person encounters a change in their surroundings.

Environment is one of the first domains where internal pressures begin to interact with the external world.

A support team arrives at a client's home early in the morning after receiving reports that the situation has escalated overnight.

Before entering the property, they can already sense the tension in the environment. Neighbours are gathered in small groups along the street, watching the house. Police vehicles are parked nearby.

Inside the home, the client is highly elevated.

They have slept poorly and appear exhausted yet intensely agitated. Loud shouting can be heard before the workers even make contact. Objects have been thrown, and the living space shows signs of recent disruption.

Attempts to engage are met with refusal. The client is distrustful and unwilling to take prescribed medication. Verbal threats are made intermittently, not always directed at a specific person but reflecting the intensity of the internal distress being experienced.

From the outside, the behaviour may appear sudden, aggressive, or deliberately confrontational.

However, the surrounding environment has already placed considerable strain on the behaviour chain. Ongoing conflict with neighbours, repeated police involvement, sleep deprivation, and heightened surveillance from others in the community have created a setting in which the client feels exposed, threatened, and overwhelmed.

In this context, behaviour becomes the visible expression of accumulated environmental pressure rather than a reaction to a single moment.

As the workers move into the home, one of them notices a familiar tightening in their chest.

The raised voices, the sense of unpredictability, and the visible distress in the environment begin to activate memories that are not immediately conscious but deeply felt.

Although professionally experienced, the worker has a personal history shaped by exposure to domestic and family violence during childhood. Situations involving shouting, threats, or loss of control can trigger an internal stress response long before thought occurs.

In this moment, the worker's own behaviour chain is also under strain.

Their interpretation of risk becomes heightened. Their expectation of escalation increases. The urge to withdraw or regain control of the situation intensifies.

Two workers in the same environment may therefore respond very differently.

One may remain grounded and able to engage therapeutically. Another may feel internally overwhelmed, leading to communication that is more directive, urgent, or defensive than intended.

The interaction between these behavioural chains can subtly influence the direction of the situation. Without awareness or support, the worker's internal response may unintentionally contribute to further escalation, despite their intention to stabilise the client.

Situations such as this illustrate how behavioural change is rarely driven by a single influence.

Multiple domains within the behaviour chain may already be under strain before support workers become involved. Environmental pressure, disrupted sleep, perceived threat, and prior experiences can all intensify the client's internal state. At the same time, workers bring their own histories, interpretations, and emotional responses into the interaction.

When these chains meet, the potential for escalation can increase if the pressure within either chain remains unrecognised. Behaviour that appears sudden or deliberate may instead reflect the cumulative effect of interacting influences that have been building over time.

Understanding the Behaviour Chain Principle encourages a broader view of these moments. Rather than focusing solely on the behaviour that becomes visible, attention can shift toward the underlying pressures shaping the interaction. This awareness creates opportunities for more measured responses, clearer boundaries, and safer outcomes for everyone involved.

After a period of heightened tension, mental health clinicians arrive on site.

They take time to observe the environment before attempting to intervene. The atmosphere remains charged, but their approach is measured and deliberate.

Rather than immediately directing the situation, the clinicians begin by acknowledging the client's distress. Their communication is calm, paced, and grounded. They listen without reinforcing threatening language and maintain clear boundaries about what can and cannot occur safely.

Gradually, the tone of the interaction begins to shift.

The client's voice lowers. Physical agitation becomes less pronounced. The clinicians are able to move closer and eventually enter the home, continuing to provide reassurance while supporting the client to regain a sense of control.

As the situation stabilises, the external environment also changes.

Neighbours disperse. Police reduce their presence and prepare to leave. The visible pressure surrounding the home decreases, allowing the client's internal state to settle further.

With support, the client agrees to take prescribed medication.

Support workers, who had earlier experienced their own stress responses, are given time to step back, debrief, and regroup before re-engaging in care.

In this moment, the behaviour chain does not break.

Instead, the strain within multiple links is gradually reduced through validation, structured boundaries, and consistent therapeutic engagement.

This outcome illustrates how the behaviour chain can be influenced not only by escalating pressures but also by timely, skilled intervention.

When clinicians responded with calm observation, validation, and clear therapeutic boundaries, they began to reduce strain across multiple domains of influence. The external environment became less threatening, expectations shifted, and emotional intensity gradually decreased.

In these moments, behaviour does not need to progress to further crisis.

Instead, the chain can regain stability as the person experiences increased safety, predictability, and containment. The interaction between individuals, services, and surroundings becomes a protective factor rather than an additional source of pressure.

Understanding the Behaviour Chain Principle in this way highlights the importance of early recognition, relational consistency, and structured responses. Behavioural escalation is not always inevitable. With awareness and coordinated support, the pressures within the chain can be eased before the fragile link gives way.

Environmental pressure does not only influence behaviour in moments of obvious crisis.

The same behavioural mechanisms are present in everyday situations, often in quieter and less visible ways. While acute environments may produce rapid escalation, more subtle settings can gradually shape how a person thinks, feels, and responds over time.

Understanding environment as a domain of influence within the behaviour chain therefore requires attention to both extremes. The intensity may differ, but the underlying process remains consistent.

A team meeting is scheduled for late afternoon after a long and demanding workday.

Most staff arrive already fatigued, carrying the mental load of competing tasks and unfinished responsibilities.

The meeting room is warm and slightly overcrowded. Conversations overlap as people settle into their seats. A supervisor begins outlining changes to upcoming routines, speaking quickly in an effort to cover several points within a limited time.

One staff member, who has been feeling increasingly overwhelmed in recent weeks, notices a sense of tension building internally. Although the information being shared is not directly critical, the environment feels pressured and difficult to process. They begin to withdraw from discussion and contribute less than usual.

Others may later read this withdrawal as disengagement or lack of motivation.

However, subtle environmental factors that accumulated quietly throughout the interaction shaped the behaviour. Fatigue, sensory discomfort, perceived expectations, and cognitive overload have all placed strain on the behaviour chain.

In situations such as this, behavioural change may be less visible but still real.

Reduced participation, avoidance, or irritability can emerge gradually as environmental pressure increases, even in the absence of overt conflict.

Environmental influences do not need to be extreme to shape behaviour. Often, it is the cumulative effect of small pressures that alters how a person engages, communicates, or responds over time.

Reflection: Noticing Environment in Your Own Practice

Think of a shift, a session, or an interaction that felt harder than usual before anything significant had happened.

Something in the room felt different.

The atmosphere carried a weight that was difficult to name.

Without pressing for an explanation, consider the following.

What was present in the environment before the interaction began?

Noise. Disruption. A change in routine. The presence or absence of a familiar person. Something unresolved from an earlier part of the day.

How did that environmental pressure shape your own internal state as you entered the interaction?

And how might it have been shaping the internal state of the person you were supporting?

This reflection is not about assigning cause.

It is about developing the habit of reading the environment before reading the behaviour.

The environment is always speaking.

The question is whether we have learned to listen to it.

Closing: Environment as the First Link

Environment does not cause behaviour directly.

It sets the conditions under which the chain begins to move.

The same person, in a different environment, may respond entirely differently.

The same worker, on a different day, may find the same situation manageable or overwhelming depending on what they brought through the door.

This is not inconsistency.

It is the chain responding to its conditions.

Understanding environment as the first link in the chain shifts the focus from the person to the system surrounding them.

It asks not only: what is this person doing?

But: what is this environment doing to this person?

That shift in question changes what becomes visible.

And what becomes visible determines what becomes possible.

In the next chapter, we follow the chain to its second link.

Because once the environment has placed its pressure on the chain, something happens inside the person experiencing it.

They begin to make meaning of what is occurring around them.

This is where interpretation begins.

Environment does not determine behaviour in isolation.

Rather, it provides the setting in which internal experiences begin to interact with external reality. In some situations, environmental pressure may be intense and highly visible. In others, it may accumulate quietly, influencing engagement, communication, and emotional regulation in more subtle ways.

Across this spectrum, the behaviour chain remains active.

Sleep deprivation, perceived threat, sensory discomfort, social expectation, and relational tension can all place varying degrees of strain on the links. Whether the outcome is crisis escalation, gradual withdrawal, or successful stabilisation often depends on how these pressures are recognised and managed within the moment.

Understanding environment as a domain of influence encourages a broader and more compassionate view of behavioural change. It reminds us that what appears sudden on the surface may have been building through a series of environmental interactions long before behaviour became visible.

However, environment alone does not explain why two people can experience the same situation and respond in quite different ways.

To understand this difference, we must look more closely at how individuals interpret what is happening around them.

This is where the next link in the behaviour chain begins to take shape.

CHAPTER THREE

Interpretation

How Events Become Personal Meaning

Interpretation is the process through which external events are translated into personal meaning. It is immediate, often unconscious, and happens before conscious thought has had time to organise itself.

It is the point in the behaviour chain where what is happening around a person becomes filtered through their internal systems. These systems include cognitive beliefs, emotional memory, physiological state, past learning, and current psychological readiness.

Because these influences operate simultaneously, interpretation is rarely neutral or purely rational.

A situation may appear straightforward from the outside yet carry vastly different meaning for the individual experiencing it. In this way, interpretation acts as a convergence point within the behaviour chain, shaping how subsequent emotional activation, expectation, and behavioural response begin to form.

A training room is filled with people preparing to become support workers.

Within the group are individuals with varied backgrounds. Some are new to the sector, while others bring lived experience of mental health challenges and personal recovery.

For some participants, the training material feels validating and empowering.

They recognise elements of their own journey in the discussion and feel motivated to use that understanding to support others.

For others, the same content activates discomfort.

Hearing descriptions of behavioural escalation, crisis situations, or trauma-informed care may trigger memories or emotional responses that are not immediately visible to those around them.

Although everyone is sitting in the same room, the interpretation of the learning environment differs. Individual recovery stage, emotional regulation capacity, and readiness to revisit past experiences all shape the meaning assigned to the material.

Participants who have developed greater insight into their own behaviour chains may be better able to notice rising internal pressure and take steps to remain regulated. Others may feel overwhelmed, withdraw from engagement, or question their suitability for the role.

In this way, interpretation influences not only how information is received, but how individuals respond to themselves within the moment.

Recognising personal domains of influence, including emotional load, past experience, and current psychological state, becomes essential in maintaining stability within the behaviour chain while undertaking support roles.

The content did not change.

The internal pressure within each person's behaviour chain did.

A woman receives a short text message from a close friend cancelling plans they had arranged earlier in the week. They have known each other for years, and plans between them are rarely cancelled.

The message is brief and offers no explanation.

"We'll have to catch up another time."

Objectively, the situation is simple. Plans have changed.

However, the meaning assigned to the message begins to shift internally.

She rereads the words several times. The lack of detail feels weighted. She wonders whether she has done something wrong. Thoughts begin to organise around perceived rejection. Emotional discomfort follows quickly, accompanied by a sense of unease that is difficult to explain.

Later that day, she responds more abruptly than usual when the friend contacts her again. The interaction becomes tense. From the outside, the reaction may appear disproportionate to the situation.

Yet the behavioural response did not begin with the text message alone.

It began with the interpretation formed in the moments after reading it.

Past experiences of exclusion, current stress levels, and underlying expectations about relationships all influenced the meaning assigned to the event. The environment presented information. Interpretation shaped the personal reality that followed.

The message did not create the reaction.

The meaning assigned to the message began the chain.

A man finishes a long shift after several nights of poor sleep. He has been covering extra hours after a colleague resigned suddenly.

He has been managing increased workload, irregular meals, and ongoing tension within his team. By the time he arrives home, his concentration feels reduced and his tolerance for minor stress is noticeably lower.

While preparing to rest, he notices a message from his manager requesting a brief discussion the following morning. The message is neutral in tone and contains no suggestion of concern or urgency.

However, in his fatigued state, the meaning assigned to the message shifts quickly.

He begins to anticipate criticism or disciplinary action. Thoughts become increasingly negative and difficult to interrupt. His body responds with restlessness and heightened arousal, making it harder to settle or sleep.

By the next day, he enters the workplace already tense and defensive. His communication style becomes abrupt, and he withdraws from collaborative interaction. Colleagues may interpret his behaviour as irritability or lack of professionalism.

Yet the behavioural change did not originate solely from the message itself.

Sleep deprivation, physical exhaustion, and accumulated stress influenced how the situation was interpreted. The physiological state of the individual shaped the meaning assigned to the event, which in turn altered emotional activation and behavioural response.

Interpretation is not only shaped by experience and belief.

It is also influenced by the condition of the body carrying the behaviour chain.

Interpretation does not always feel like a conscious decision or a conscious process. In many situations, meaning is assigned automatically, influenced by past experiences, emotional readiness, and current physical or psychological state.

When interpretation occurs rapidly, a person may experience a shift in feeling before they have fully understood why. Discomfort, tension, defensiveness, or withdrawal can emerge without a clear awareness of what has triggered the change. From the outside, behaviour may appear unexpected or disproportionate. Internally, however, the response can feel justified or necessary.

Developing awareness of interpretation within the behaviour chain can create opportunities for earlier regulation. When individuals begin to recognise how they assign meaning to situations, they may be better able to pause, reflect, and consider alternative explanations. This does not eliminate emotional response, but it can reduce the likelihood of behaviour escalating to a point where control feels lost.

Support workers, carers, and professionals can also benefit from understanding interpretation as a domain of influence. Recognising that behaviour is shaped by perceived meaning rather than objective reality alone can encourage more measured responses, clearer communication, and greater empathy in moments of tension.

In this way, interpretation becomes not only a point of vulnerability within the behaviour chain, but also a potential point of intervention.

Reflection: Noticing Interpretation in Real Time

Think of a recent situation in which your emotional response felt stronger than you expected.

It may have involved a conversation, a change of plans, a request you did not feel ready for, or an interaction that left you unsettled afterwards.

Without analysing the situation in detail, pause and consider the following.

What did the moment come to mean for you at the time?

What did you assume was happening or about to happen?

How did your body respond as this meaning began to form?

Did your behaviour shift quickly, or did it change gradually?

Looking back now, what other factors, in the present moment or from your history, might have shaped the meaning you assigned to that situation?

This reflection is not about judging your reaction.

It is about recognising how interpretation influences emotional activation and behavioural response.

Awareness of this process does not remove distress or prevent all behavioural change.

However, it can create a small but important space between experience and action.

Within that space, regulation becomes more possible.

Closing: Interpretation as the Turning Point

Interpretation represents a critical turning point within the behaviour chain.

It is the stage at which external events begin to take on personal meaning, shaping emotional activation and influencing the direction of behavioural response. Although situations may appear similar on the surface, the meanings assigned to them can vary widely between individuals.

This process is rarely conscious.

Interpretation is influenced by accumulated experiences, emotional learning, physiological state, and perceived safety within the moment. As a result, behavioural change often reflects not only what is happening now, but also what the present situation connects to internally.

Developing awareness of interpretation can increase a person's capacity to pause and consider alternative perspectives. This awareness does not eliminate emotional response, nor does it prevent all escalation. However, it can reduce the speed at which pressure builds within the behaviour chain and create opportunities for earlier regulation.

To understand why certain interpretations, feel immediate, intense, or difficult to challenge, we need to open a door that most people sense but rarely examine directly.

The emotional archive. The accumulated record of everything that has ever happened to us, and the felt sense it left behind.

CHAPTER FOUR

Memory

The Emotional Archive

Not all responses to the present moment are created in the present moment.

Experiences accumulate over time.

Some are processed, understood, and gradually integrated into a person's sense of self. Others remain stored in ways that continue to influence perception, emotional activation, and behavioural response long after the original event has passed.

Memory acts as an emotional archive within the behaviour chain.

It holds the residue of past interactions, learned expectations about safety or threat, and the personal meanings that were formed during earlier stages of life.

In certain situations, a current event may resemble something that has been experienced before. The similarity may be obvious, or it may be subtle and difficult to articulate. A tone of voice, a pattern of communication, a loss of control, or a perceived rejection can activate memories that shape how the present moment is understood.

When this occurs, behaviour may appear to be a reaction to what is happening now.

In reality, experiences that have already shaped the person's emotional landscape may be driving the response.

Understanding memory as a domain of influence within the behaviour chain helps explain why reactions can feel immediate, intense, or difficult to regulate. The past is not simply remembered. At times, it is re-experienced through the meaning assigned to the present.

Memory is not a single, unified system.

It does not function like a recording that can be played back accurately on demand.

It is better understood as a collection of systems, each storing different kinds of experience in different ways.

Some memories are explicit, conscious, declarative, able to be described in words.

A person can recall an event, place it in time, and speak about it with some degree of coherence.

These are the memories most people think of when the word memory is used.

But within the behaviour chain, it is a different kind of memory that often carries the most weight.

Implicit memory, sometimes called emotional or procedural memory, stores experience not as a narrative but as a felt sense.

A physiological response.

A pattern of expectation.

A way of being in the body when certain conditions are present.

Implicit memory does not always announce itself.

It does not say: this reminds me of something that happened before.

It simply activates.

A person may find themselves suddenly tense without knowing why.

Suddenly guarded in a situation that appears, by any objective measure, to be safe.

Suddenly certain that something is about to go wrong, even in the absence of any clear evidence.

These responses are not irrational.

They are the product of an archive that has been carefully and quietly assembled across a lifetime of experience. An archive that is doing exactly what it was designed to do.

Protecting the person from harm it has learned to anticipate.

A woman in her late thirties has been accessing community mental health support for several years.

She is articulate, insightful, and has developed a strong working relationship with her support coordinator.

One afternoon, the coordinator arrives for a scheduled visit and mentions, in passing, that they will be going on leave in three weeks.

The information is delivered warmly, with care, and with reassurance that cover arrangements are in place.

The coordinator notices, however, that something changes in the room as the words land.

The woman's posture shifts almost imperceptibly.

Her responses become slightly shorter.

A quality of engagement that was present at the beginning of the visit begins to withdraw.

By the end of the session, she is polite but distant.

The coordinator leaves feeling uncertain about what changed and why.

What the coordinator could not fully see was the archive being accessed in the moment the word leave was spoken.

The woman's history includes multiple experiences of significant people departing without adequate notice or care.

A parent who left during childhood.

A previous support worker whose sudden resignation was communicated by a manager, not by the worker themselves.

A close friendship that ended abruptly and without explanation.

Each of these experiences has been stored, not only as a conscious memory that can be described, but as a pattern.

A learned anticipation about what happens when people say they are going away.

The coordinator's leave, offered with full transparency and genuine care, was filtered through that archive.

And what emerged from that filtering was not the message that was sent.

It was a message shaped by everything the archive had learned to expect.

The relationship between memory and interpretation is not simply sequential.

Memory does not wait politely for interpretation to complete before it contributes.

It is active within the interpretive process itself.

When a person encounters a new situation, the brain moves rapidly through its archive, seeking patterns, comparing the present with what has been stored, forming a sense of familiarity or unfamiliarity, safety, or threat.

This process is largely unconscious.

It is also remarkably fast.

By the time a person has consciously registered what is happening around them, the archive has already been consulted.

The emotional tone of the response has already begun to form.

This is why telling someone that their emotional response is disproportionate to the situation is rarely effective.

From the outside, the current situation may appear manageable and unthreatening.

From the inside, the archive has already found a match, and that match is informing the experience of the present in ways that cannot be easily overridden by rational assessment.

The body is responding to what it has learned, not only to what is happening.

Early experiences occupy a place within the emotional archive.

The memories formed during childhood and adolescence, particularly those formed within significant relationships and within contexts of stress, unpredictability, or harm, tend to carry unusual weight within the behaviour chain.

This is not arbitrary.

The brain is most actively developing its foundational patterns of response during these early years.

The experiences absorbed during this period do not simply add to the archive.

They help shape its architecture.

They influence how the nervous system learns to calibrate threat.

How the body learns to respond when safety feels uncertain.

What kinds of relationships come to feel familiar.

What kinds of interactions trigger the deepest and most rapid responses.

A child who grew up in an environment where adult behaviour was unpredictable may develop an archive that is finely tuned to detecting the early signals of instability in others.

A child whose early needs were consistently unmet may develop an archive that expects disappointment before it has occurred.

A child who experienced harm within a relationship that should have offered safety may develop an archive that treats closeness itself as a potential source of danger.

None of this is pathology.
All of it is adaptation.

The archive assembled in childhood was assembled in response to a real environment.

It was built to protect.

It was built to help the person navigate a world that offered its own challenges.

The difficulty is that the archive, once assembled, does not automatically update when the world changes.

An adult who now exists in a genuinely safer environment may still carry an archive calibrated for a more dangerous one.

And that archive will continue to shape interpretation, understanding, and emotional response. Not because the person is choosing to live in the past, but because the past is not finished shaping the present.

A young man has been living in supported accommodation for eight months.

He is twenty-two years old and has spent the majority of his adolescence moving between placements, family arrangements that did not hold, and periods of homelessness.

The support team working with him are experienced and committed.

They have taken considerable care to establish clear expectations, consistent routines, and a relational environment that communicates safety and predictability.

By most observable measures, the placement is going well.

Then, one evening, one of the key support workers fails to show up for a scheduled shift.

There is a reason, a family emergency, and a replacement worker is arranged.

The communication is handled as well as it can be in the circumstances.

The young man's response, however, is significant.

He becomes withdrawn and refuses to engage with the replacement worker.

Over the following days, his behaviour shifts in ways the team finds difficult to understand.

He becomes harder to reach.

Old patterns of resistance that had largely settled begin to resurface.

His trust in the team, which has been carefully built over months, appears to have destabilised overnight.

The team discusses what happened.

They are bewildered, because the incident, a single missed shift handled with appropriate communication, does not seem proportionate to the response.

But the response is not to the missed shift.

The response is to what the missed shift has activated within the archive.

Eight months of consistent experience has not yet been sufficient to overwrite the weight of years in which inconsistency was the norm.

The archive's pattern, that people leave, arrangements fail, and safety does not hold, has been activated by a single piece of evidence that matches what has always been expected.

One data point, filtered through an archive assembled across years of contrary experience, has temporarily undone eight months of careful relationship-building.

This is not failure.

This is the behaviour chain working exactly as it is designed to work.

For support workers and clinicians, understanding the role of memory within the behaviour chain changes what patience means.

Patience is not simply waiting for a person to respond differently.

It is the sustained provision of experiences that are inconsistent with what the archive has learned to expect.

Every interaction that proceeds differently from what the archive has anticipated is a small piece of new information.

Every consistent, trustworthy, boundaried response is a quiet challenge to a pattern that was assembled in a different environment.

This process is slow.

It is non-linear.

It does not proceed in an orderly direction from damage toward recovery.

It moves forward and backward.

It accelerates and stalls.

It can appear, after months of progress, to have reversed entirely, only to re-emerge, sometimes within days, with greater stability than was present before the disruption.

This is the nature of working with memory within the behaviour chain.

The archive does not update through instruction.

It updates through experience.

And the most powerful experiences available, the ones that carry the most weight against the patterns already stored, are not dramatic interventions or clinical breakthroughs.

They are the unremarkable, repeated, consistent moments of being treated with predictability and care.

The worker who shows up when they said they would.

The team that responds to difficulty without withdrawing support.

The environment that holds its shape even when the person within it is testing whether it will.

These are the experiences that, over time, begin to rewrite what the archive expects.

Memory also operates within the worker's chain.

A support worker who grew up in an environment shaped by conflict or instability will carry an archive that responds to certain situations with a speed and intensity that may surprise them.

The sound of raised voices.

The quality of a silence that precedes escalation.

The feeling of being responsible for managing someone else's emotional state.

These are not professional responses to a professional situation.

They are the archive activating patterns that were laid down before the worker ever entered the sector.

A worker who can recognise this, who can notice when their response to a situation belongs more to their archive than to the present moment, has access to a quality of self-awareness that changes what is possible in the interaction.

Not because the archive disappears.

But because awareness of its operation creates the small but significant space between activation and response.

In that space, the worker can choose.

Reflection: Listening to the Archive

Think of a situation, recent or from your past, in which your emotional response arrived faster or with more intensity than you would have expected.

Perhaps it was a moment in which you felt suddenly defensive.

Suddenly certain that someone was about to let you down.

Suddenly overwhelmed by a situation that, from the outside, might have appeared manageable.

Without pressing for an explanation, sit with the following questions.

What did the situation remind you of, even faintly?

Is there an earlier experience, perhaps from childhood, perhaps from a relationship or a previous role, which carries a similar emotional shape?

When you felt the response arrive, where did you feel it in your body?

Was it a tightening? A withdrawal? A sudden alertness?

Did you act from that response, or were you able to notice it before acting?

And looking back, what different factors, both in the present moment and from your past, might have contributed to the strength of your response?

This reflection is not an invitation to excavate painful history.

It is an invitation to develop a listening relationship with the archive.

The archive is not an enemy.

It is a record of everything a person has survived and learned.

But when it speaks, it is worth knowing that it is speaking, so that its voice can be heard with awareness rather than simply obeyed.

Closing: Memory as a Living Influence

Memory is not the past sitting quietly behind us.

It is an active presence within the behaviour chain, consulting, comparing, anticipating, and shaping the meaning assigned to every new experience.

It explains why the same situation can feel entirely different to two people standing in it.

Why a response can feel immediate and certain before thought has occurred.

Why progress in a support relationship can appear to reverse overnight, and why that reversal, while painful, is not the undoing of everything that came before.

Understanding memory as a domain of influence within the behaviour chain does not mean excavating every person's history before support can begin.

It means holding an awareness that history is always present, in the quality of attention someone brings to an interaction, in the speed and intensity of their emotional response, in the patterns of behaviour that seem most deeply entrenched.

And it means recognising that the most powerful thing a support worker, a clinician, or a care team can offer is not always a new technique or a refined intervention.

Sometimes the most powerful thing is simply this.

A consistent, trustworthy presence.

Offered repeatedly, without condition, across enough time that the archive begins, slowly, imperfectly, but genuinely, to expect something different.

In the next chapter, we follow the chain to its next link.

Because once memory has shaped the way a situation is interpreted, the person must arrive at some working sense of what is actually happening.

This is the link of understanding.

And it is where the internal world of the chain begins to crystallise into something that will determine how behaviour finally forms.

CHAPTER FIVE

Understanding

Making Sense of What Is Happening

Memory does not simply store the past.

It carries it forward.

And when the past is carried into the present, it does not arrive labelled or explained.

It arrives as feeling.

As a shift in the body.

As a sudden certainty about what a situation means before thought has occurred.

This is where the next link in the behaviour chain begins to take shape.

Once a person has interpreted an event and memory has contributed its weight to that interpretation, something must happen next.

The person must make sense of what is occurring around them.

They must arrive at some working understanding of the situation.

Understanding is distinct from interpretation. Where interpretation is the immediate, often wordless assignment of meaning, understanding is the conclusion that forms in its wake. It is the working story a person constructs about what is happening, why it is happening, and what it is likely to mean for them.

It does not require insight or awareness.

It simply refers to where a person has landed, consciously or not, in their sense of the situation.

Sometimes that conclusion is accurate.

Sometimes it is not.

But accurate or not, it shapes everything that follows.

A young woman is being supported by a disability support worker during a routine medical appointment.

The appointment has been on the calendar for several weeks. She has mentioned, more than once, that she finds medical settings hard.

The worker has reminded her of it gently and prepared her as much as possible.

On the morning of the appointment, however, the environment is already strained.

The woman slept poorly. Her usual routine has broken down. The waiting room at the clinic is crowded and loud, with fluorescent lighting and overlapping conversations pressing in from every direction.

The doctor enters the room and speaks quickly.

The appointment is efficient and professional, but the pace does not allow for questions. Information is given. Instructions are provided. The consultation ends.

As they leave, the support worker notices a change.

The woman has become quiet. Her posture has shifted. She is walking more quickly than usual and has stopped making eye contact.

Later, back at home, she refuses to engage with the support worker and asks to be left alone.

The worker wonders whether something was said during the appointment that caused offence.

But the behaviour did not begin with offence.

It began with understanding.

During the appointment, the woman had reached a conclusion about what was happening around her.

Interpretation and memory had filtered the noise, the pace, the clinical environment, and the rapid delivery of information.

The understanding she arrived at was not that she had attended a routine appointment.

It was that the appointment had overwhelmed her, left her unheard, and outpaced what she could manage.

That understanding, formed quietly and without words, became the lens through which the rest of the interaction was experienced.

Withdrawal was not a response to the appointment itself.

It was a response to what the appointment had come to mean.

Understanding is shaped by several influences operating at once.

The first is the information actually available in the moment.

What can be seen, heard, and sensed.

What has been said and what has been left unsaid.

The second is the interpretation already formed.

Because understanding follows interpretation, it is built on a foundation that may already be altered by past experience, emotional state, and the meaning assigned to events.

The third is cognitive capacity in the moment.

A person who is fatigued, overwhelmed, in pain, or under significant stress will often reach different conclusions than they would in a calmer state.

This is not a failure of intelligence.

It is the natural effect of cognitive load on the process of making sense.

When cognitive capacity is reduced, understanding tends to simplify.

Complex situations become flatter.

Nuance disappears.

The world narrows to what feels most immediately true, most familiar, or most threatening.

This narrowing is a feature of how human beings manage overwhelming information.

But it can also place significant strain on the behaviour chain.

A support worker arrives for an afternoon shift to find that the usual team leader is absent.

In their place is a worker they do not know well, someone who joined the team recently and has a different communication style.

The shift briefing is delivered quickly.

Several changes to the client's plan have been made without prior notice to the worker, and the explanation offered is brief.

The worker nods and begins the shift.

But internally, something is forming.

They do not have enough information to understand why the changes were made.

Their experience of the briefing has already been filtered through interpretation, shaped by the absence of the familiar team leader, the unfamiliar face, and the rushed communication.

The understanding they arrive at is not that changes were made for clinical reasons.

It is that their input is not valued.

That something is happening in the team that they are not being told about.

That they are being managed rather than supported.

None of this may be true.

But understanding does not require accuracy.

It requires only that a conclusion has been reached.

For the remainder of the shift, the worker's engagement is altered.

Their communication with the client becomes slightly more mechanical.

Their willingness to raise concerns decreases.

Pressure has moved through the chain, not because of what was said, but because of what was understood.

Understanding as a link in the behaviour chain carries special significance for support workers and clinicians.

When working alongside someone whose understanding of their situation is limited, distorted by past experience, or shaped by cognitive or psychological factors, it can be tempting to simply correct the conclusion.

To offer the facts.

To explain what is actually happening.

But understanding does not respond well to correction alone.

A person who has concluded that they are under threat will not immediately feel safe because someone tells them they are.

A person who has understood an interaction as rejection will not immediately feel accepted because someone explains that no rejection was intended.

Understanding sits downstream from interpretation and memory.

To shift the understanding, it is often necessary to first acknowledge what the person has concluded, and to recognise the internal logic that led them there.

This is not agreement.

It is validation.

When a support worker says, in effect, I can see why this felt that way to you, they are not confirming that the conclusion was accurate.

They are creating the conditions under which a different understanding might become possible.

Without that step, offering facts can feel like further evidence that the person has not been heard.

And a person who does not feel heard is unlikely to reach a new understanding easily.

Reflection: Noticing Understanding in the Moment

Think of a recent situation in which you formed a strong sense of what was happening, only to discover later that your understanding was incomplete or incorrect.

It may have been a conversation that left you feeling dismissed, a decision that seemed to exclude you, or a change that appeared to signal something significant.

Without judging the conclusion you reached, consider the following:

What information did you have available at the time?

What information was missing?

How did your interpretation of the situation, and perhaps a memory connected to it, shape the understanding you arrived at?

How did that understanding influence your behaviour during or after the event?

What would have needed to happen for a different understanding to form?

This reflection is not about deciding whether your conclusion was right or wrong.

It is about noticing that understanding is a process.

One that is shaped by what we bring to a situation, not only by what the situation contains.

Awareness of this process does not prevent misunderstanding from occurring.

But it can create the space to pause and ask:

Is this what is actually happening, or is this what I have concluded is happening?

That pause, however brief, can change the direction of the chain.

Closing: Understanding as a Turning Point

Understanding is not the same as knowledge.

It is the personal sense a person makes of what is happening around them, formed rapidly and often without conscious awareness.

When understanding is clear, proportionate, and grounded in accurate information, it can stabilise the behaviour chain.

The situation feels manageable. Expectations are reasonable. Emotional response is calibrated to what is actually occurring.

But when understanding is shaped by incomplete information, distorted by past experience, or narrowed by cognitive load, it can place significant strain on the chain.

The situation feels different than it is.

The response that follows reflects not reality, but the meaning assigned to it.

For support workers, carers, and clinicians, recognising how understanding forms within the people they support is one of the most practical skills available.

It shifts the question from what is wrong with this person to what has this person concluded, and what led them there.

That shift in question changes the quality of support that becomes possible.

Understanding is not fixed.

It can change when a person feels safe enough to consider a different interpretation.

When the environment settles enough for cognitive capacity to return.

When someone alongside them offers not correction, but validation.

These are the moments when the chain can be strengthened before the fragile link gives way.

In the next chapter, we explore what happens within the chain once understanding has formed.

Because understanding does not exist in isolation.

It activates something.
And what it activates will shape everything that follows.

CHAPTER SIX

Emotion

Activation, Regulation, and Dysregulation

Understanding does not sit still.

Once a person has made sense of what is happening around them, once they have arrived at a conclusion about the meaning of a situation, something shifts inside the body.

That shift is emotion.

Emotion is not a thought.

It is not a decision.

It is not something a person chooses to experience.

It is the body's response to meaning.

When a situation has been interpreted, filtered through memory, and understood in one way, the nervous system responds to that understanding as though it were fact.

It does not wait for verification.

It does not pause to consider alternative explanations.

It responds to what has been concluded, not to what is objectively occurring.

This is why emotion can feel so immediate.

So certain.

So difficult to reason with from the outside.

The conclusion came first.

The emotion followed.

And by the time the emotion is visible to others, the chain has already been building for some time.

A man in his mid-forties lives alone and is supported by a disability support team several times each week.

He values his routine deeply. Predictability gives him a sense of safety that is not easily replaced by reassurance or explanation.

One afternoon, a worker arrives twenty minutes late.

No message has been sent. No explanation has come.

By the time the worker knocks at the door, the man has already moved through several links in his chain.

He has noticed the disruption and assigned it meaning.

Memory has contributed. Previous experiences of unreliability, of people not showing up, of plans falling through without warning.

An understanding has formed: something is wrong. The support cannot be trusted. The day is already lost.

And now, as the door opens, emotion arrives.

It does not arrive gently.

It arrives as agitation, sharpness, a voice that is louder than the worker expected and a body that is turned away from the room.

The worker, who had a minor car issue and had intended to explain, finds themselves immediately on the back foot.

They did not see the twenty minutes of internal chain-building that preceded their arrival.

They only see the emotion that greets them at the door.

From the outside, the response can seem disproportionate.

From the inside, it is the only response that makes sense.

Emotion serves a purpose.

This is important to understand, particularly for those working in support roles.

Emotion is not dysfunction.

It is not weakness.

It is not manipulation, even when it feels that way from the outside.

Emotion is the body preparing to respond to what it believes is happening.

Fear prepares the body to flee or to freeze.

Anger prepares the body to push back, to defend, to create distance.

Sadness signals loss and draws the person inward.

Anxiety anticipates a threat that has not yet fully arrived.

Each of these states has a function.

Each has evolved to help human beings navigate situations that feel threatening, uncertain, or beyond their control.

The difficulty is not that emotion exists.

The difficulty arises when the emotional response is no longer matched to the actual situation.

When the nervous system responds to a twenty-minute delay as though it were abandonment.

When a change of plan triggers a response more suited to genuine danger.

When a neutral tone of voice is experienced as contempt.

In these moments, the emotion itself is not wrong.

It is responding accurately to the conclusion that has formed.

The understanding may be inaccurate.

But the emotion is doing exactly what it is designed to do.

Emotional regulation is the capacity to experience an emotional state without being entirely governed by it.

It does not mean suppressing emotion.

It does not mean performing calm when distress is present.

It means having enough internal space between the feeling and the response to make a considered choice about what happens next.

For some people, this capacity is well developed.

They can notice a strong emotional response, recognise it as such, and adjust their behaviour accordingly.

They can feel angry without acting on the anger in ways they would later regret.

They can feel anxious without allowing the anxiety to dictate their decisions.

For others, this capacity is more limited.

Early experiences that did not allow for safe emotional expression may have shaped it.

By environments where emotion was a source of danger rather than connection.

By a nervous system that has learned, over many years, to treat uncertainty as threat.

In these situations, emotional dysregulation is not a character flaw.

It is a learned response to a world that once required it.

A support worker has been providing care to a young woman for several months.

The relationship has developed steadily. Trust has formed. Progress has been visible.

Then a change in rostering means that another worker will take over three of the weekly sessions.

The change is necessary, clearly explained, and accompanied by a transition plan.

Despite this, the young woman's behaviour shifts noticeably in the days that follow.

She becomes withdrawn during sessions.

She cancels two appointments without explanation.

When she does attend, she is present physically but emotionally distant.

The support worker who remains in her roster tries to engage with what has changed.

The young woman finds it difficult to explain.

She knows, intellectually, that the change is reasonable.

She knows the new worker is qualified and kind.

But understanding has already been filtered through memory.

Early experiences of significant people leaving without warning.

Of transitions that were not handled with care.

Of stability that did not hold.

The emotion sitting behind this reaction is not about the rostering change.

It is a response to what this rostering change has come to represent.

The body does not distinguish easily between a past loss and a present one.

It responds to the emotional memory as much as to the current event.

And when the emotional response is this connected to history, regulation becomes more difficult.

The gap between feeling and behaviour narrows.

The chain moves quickly toward the fragile link.

For support workers, understanding emotional activation and dysregulation changes the way a situation can be approached.

When a client becomes emotionally elevated, the instinct can be to address the behaviour directly.

To name what is happening.

To explain. To correct. To redirect.

But a person in a state of emotional dysregulation is not fully available to reason.

The part of the brain most involved in logical thought and considered decision-making is significantly less accessible when the nervous system is activated.

This is not a choice.

It is physiology.

What the person needs in that moment is not information.

It is safety.

Safety is communicated through tone before it is communicated through words.

Through a body that is calm and unhurried.

Through a voice that does not rise to meet the distress.

Through proximity that respects rather than crowds.

Through responses that acknowledge rather than dismiss.

A person cannot be regulated by someone who is dysregulated themselves.

This is one of the most practical and important truths in the entire behaviour chain.

A worker who enters an elevated situation already carrying their own emotional activation, from a hard shift, a strained relationship, an unresolved conflict in the team, will find it significantly harder to offer the kind of co-regulation that can stabilise the chain.

The worker's own emotional state is not separate from the interaction.

It is part of it.

Reflection: Noticing Emotional Activation in Yourself

Think of a recent interaction, either personal or professional, in which you noticed your emotional state shift.

It may have been a moment of unexpected irritation.
A sudden withdrawal from a conversation.

A tension in the body that arrived before you had fully understood why.

Without judging the response, consider the following:

What had you understood about the situation in the moments before the emotion arrived?

What memory or past experience might have contributed to that understanding?

Where did you feel the emotion in your body?

Did your behaviour change as a result of the emotional state you were in?

Looking back, how much space was there between the feeling and your response?

This reflection is not about assessing your emotional regulation capacity.

It is about recognising that emotion is a link in the chain, one that connects what has already happened inside the chain to what is about to happen at the end of it.

When you can begin to notice your own emotional activation, you create the possibility of making a different choice before the chain reaches its fragile point.

Closing: Emotion as Signal, Not Sentence

Emotion is not the enemy of good support.

It is a signal.

A message from the nervous system about how a situation has been understood.

About what the body believes is required.

About how far along the chain the person has already travelled.

When emotion becomes visible, in a client, in a colleague, in ourselves, it is an invitation to look earlier in the chain rather than later.

To ask not what this person is doing, but what has this person concluded, and what is their body trying to do about it.

Emotional dysregulation is not a fixed state.

It shifts with the environment, with the quality of relational connection, with the presence or absence of predictability and safety.

A person who is dysregulated in one context may find regulation far more accessible in another.

The difference is often not within the person alone.

It is in the chain of influences that surrounds them.

Understanding this does not remove the difficulty of working alongside strong emotional responses.

It does not make dysregulation easy to sit with or simple to manage.

But it changes the frame.

It shifts the focus from the behaviour that emotion produces to the meaning that emotion is communicating.

And once we can hear what the emotion is saying, we are closer to being able to respond to what is actually needed.

In the next chapter, we follow the chain to its final internal link.

Because once emotion has been activated, the person begins to anticipate.

They begin to form a sense of what is coming next.

And what they expect will shape how they behave.

CHAPTER SEVEN

Expectation

What We Anticipate Shapes What We Do

Emotion does not simply arrive and settle.

Once activated, it reaches forward.

It begins to scan the situation ahead.

To form a picture of what is coming next.

To anticipate, based on everything already held within the chain, what the next moment is likely to bring.

This is expectation.

And expectation is one of the most powerful forces within the behaviour chain.

Not because of what it tells us about the future.

But because of what it causes us to do in the present.

A person who expects to be dismissed will often speak before they are spoken to, in ways that confirm the dismissal.

A person who expects to be hurt will protect themselves before any harm has occurred.

A person who expects failure will disengage from the attempt before the outcome is known.

In each case, the behaviour that follows is not a response to what has happened.

It is a response to what the person is certain is about to happen.

The future has not yet arrived.

But the body is already preparing for it.

A teenage boy has moved into supported accommodation following a period of significant family instability.

He has experienced multiple placement breakdowns in the previous two years.

Each time, the ending has felt sudden, regardless of the explanations offered.

He is now settled in a new placement with support workers who are consistent, warm, and committed to his care.

Several weeks in, one of the workers mentions casually that they will be taking leave the following month.

The conversation is brief. The context is ordinary.

But inside the boy's chain, the mention of the worker's absence does not land as ordinary.

Environment, interpretation, and memory have already shaped the way this moment is processed.

Emotion is moving through the chain.

And now expectation begins to form.

He does not consciously decide what is coming next.

The expectation arrives as certainty.

This is how it ends.

They always leave eventually.

There is no point in continuing to trust.
In the days that follow, his behaviour shifts.

He becomes harder to engage.

He pushes against boundaries that he had previously accepted without resistance.

He begins to create distance in small ways that feel, from the outside, like deliberate testing.

He is not testing the worker.

He is preparing for an ending he is certain is coming.

Because when endings happen suddenly, being the one who withdraws first is the only form of control available.

Expectation is not passive.

It is active.

It shapes behaviour before the anticipated event has occurred.

And in doing so, it can sometimes bring about the very outcome the person feared most.

Expectation is formed from the materials already present within the chain.

What has been interpreted about the current situation.

What memory has contributed about similar situations in the past.

What has been understood about what is happening and why.

What emotion has signalled about the level of threat or safety present.

All of these influences converge in the moment before a person acts.

And from that convergence, an anticipation is formed.

Sometimes the expectation is grounded in accurate reading of the situation.

A person who has learned that a particular environment becomes unsafe at certain times of day, and who anticipates that pattern and prepares accordingly, is using expectation well.

But when expectation is shaped primarily by fear, by prior harm, or by a nervous system that has learned to anticipate the worst in order to survive it, the picture formed can be at significant odds with what is actually unfolding.

The situation in front of the person may be safe.

The people around them may be trustworthy.

The outcome may be entirely different from what has come before.

But expectation does not always wait for evidence.

A support worker has been delivering services to a woman who has had difficult experiences with previous support providers.

She has described, in team discussions, feeling unheard, managed, and dismissed by workers who did not take her preferences seriously.

The new worker is thoughtful and careful.

They communicate clearly, offer choices, and make deliberate efforts to follow the woman's lead.

Despite this, certain interactions become tense in ways the worker finds difficult to understand.

When the worker suggests, even an options-based one, the woman sometimes responds with resistance that feels out of proportion to the moment.

What is happening inside the chain is not resistance to this worker or this suggestion.

It is the activation of an expectation formed long before this worker arrived.

The expectation is not simply that this suggestion will be dismissed.

It is that this is how support works.

Suggestions become instructions.

Choice becomes an illusion.

And eventually, the person's preferences will be overridden.

The woman is not responding to what this worker is doing.

She is responding to what every previous version of this interaction has meant.

Her expectation has arrived before the worker's suggestion has finished forming.

And it is shaping her response to a situation she has, in many ways, already decided the outcome of.

For support workers, expectation presents its own challenge.

It is invisible.

A worker can observe behaviour.

They can notice emotion when it becomes expressed.

They can hear the words a person uses and respond to them.

But expectation exists just before all of this.

It operates in the fraction of a moment between the situation presenting itself and the person beginning to respond.

It cannot be seen.

It can only be inferred.

And yet, understanding that expectation is operating can change everything about how a situation is approached.

When a client's response seems disproportionate, expectation may already be at work.

When a person withdraws before anything has gone wrong, expectation may already be directing the movement.

When resistance appears in a moment that should, by any objective measure, feel manageable, expectation may already have decided the outcome.

Recognising this does not require certainty about what the person is anticipating.

It simply requires the willingness to ask a different question.

Not: why are they behaving like this?

But: what are they expecting to happen next?

That shift in question opens a different kind of conversation.

One that does not challenge the behaviour directly but instead creates space for the expectation beneath it to become visible.

When the expectation can be named, ideally by the person themselves but at times gently reflected by the worker, it loses some of its certainty.

It becomes something to consider rather than something that simply happens.

Expectation also operates within the worker's own chain.

A worker who has experienced repeated escalation with a client will often develop an expectation that the next interaction will escalate too.

That expectation changes the way they enter the interaction.

They may become more cautious.

More directive.

More focused on managing potential outcomes than on being present to what is actually occurring.

Paradoxically, this shift in the worker's behaviour, driven by their own expectation, can communicate something to the client.

The worker's tension is felt before any words are spoken.

Their bracing for difficulty can be read, by a nervous system attuned to threat, as confirmation that something difficult is indeed approaching.

Two expectations, held by two people, can meet in the space between them and create the very outcome both were anticipating.

This is why understanding expectation is not only useful for understanding client behaviour.

It is essential for understanding the role the worker plays within the interaction.

Reflection: Noticing Expectation Before It Acts

Think of a situation, recent or from your past, in which you entered an interaction already certain about how it would unfold.

Perhaps you expected conflict.

Perhaps you expected to be misunderstood.

Perhaps you expected that your effort would not be recognised, or that a particular person would respond in a way you had come to anticipate.

Without judging the expectation, consider the following:

What had already happened within your chain before you entered that interaction?

What interpretation, memory, or emotional state had contributed to the anticipation you were carrying?

Did your behaviour change because of the expectation before the anticipated event had even occurred?

Looking back, was the expectation confirmed?

And if it was, is it possible that the expectation itself played a part in shaping the outcome?

This is not about self-blame.

It is about recognising that expectation is an active force within the chain.

One that can move ahead of us into situations we have not yet fully entered.

When expectation can be noticed, even briefly, even imperfectly, there is an opportunity to pause.

To ask whether the picture being formed is one drawn from the present or carried forward from somewhere else.

That question does not always change the outcome.

But it creates space where previously there was none.

Closing: Expectation as the Final Internal Link

Expectation is where the internal world of the behaviour chain meets the edge of action.

By the time expectation has formed, the person has already moved through environment, interpretation, memory, understanding, and emotion.

Each link has contributed to the anticipation now present.

What the person expects to happen next is not random.

It is the logical conclusion of everything that has already moved through the chain.

It may not be accurate.
It may not reflect what is actually about to occur.

But to the person carrying it, it carries the weight of certainty.

And certainty, particularly certainty about threat or loss, does not wait for confirmation before it acts.

For support workers and clinicians, recognising expectation within a client's behaviour is one of the most nuanced and valuable skills available.

It requires looking not only at what a person is doing, but at what they are anticipating.

Not only at the response in front of you, but at the picture of the future being held just behind it.

When expectation can be gently acknowledged, when a worker can communicate through presence and consistency that this interaction may unfold differently than the one being anticipated, the chain can be interrupted before behaviour reaches the fragile link.

Not always.

Not immediately.

But over time, consistent experience that contradicts a harmful expectation is one of the most powerful forces available for change.

In the next chapter, we arrive at the final link.

The one that has been forming throughout this entire journey.

Behaviour.

The visible end of a chain that began long before anyone watching could see it.

CHAPTER EIGHT

Behaviour

The Visible End of the Chain

We have arrived at the end.

Not the end of the story.

The end of the chain.

Everything explored in the preceding chapters, environment, interpretation, memory, understanding, emotion, expectation, has been moving toward this point.

Quietly, often invisibly, building pressure through links that cannot always be seen from the outside.

And now, at the end of all of that internal movement, something becomes visible.

Behaviour.

The moment a person raises their voice.

Withdraws from a conversation.

Refuses a request.

Walks away.

Escalates.

Shuts down.

From the outside, behaviour often appears as though it has arrived without warning.

As though something was said or done, and a person simply reacted.

But we know now that this is not how it works.

Behaviour is never the beginning of the event.

It is the end of it.

A man in his early thirties has been living independently for two years, supported by a small team of workers who assist him with daily tasks and community access.

It is a Tuesday morning.

By any external measure, it appears to be an ordinary day.

The worker arrives on time.

The greeting is warm.

Nothing unusual has been said.

And then, within minutes, the man refuses to leave his bedroom.

He does not respond to gentle prompting.

When the worker persists, his voice rises sharply.

He states, with considerable force, that he wants the worker to leave.

The worker, who has had no prior indication that this morning would be different from any other, is caught off guard.

They feel the sting of the refusal personally, even as they try not to.

They wonder what they did wrong.

But the behaviour did not begin with the worker's arrival.

The night before, there had been a phone call from a family member that left unresolved tension.

Sleep had been fitful and insufficient.

The morning had begun with a small but significant disruption to routine. A different brand of coffee, the kind of detail that matters more than it appears to.

By the time the worker arrived, the chain had already been under strain for hours.

The greeting was warm.

The worker did nothing wrong.

But the chain did not know that.

The chain only knew that it had reached its fragile point.

And when the worker persisted with the plan for the day, that persistence became the final pressure.

Behaviour changed.

Not because of the worker.

Because of everything that had already moved through the chain before they knocked on the door.

Behaviour, when it finally appears, serves a function.

This is essential to understand.

Behaviour is not random noise at the end of a chain.

It is purposeful.

It is the person's best available response to the internal state they are in and the situation they believe they are facing.

Sometimes that purpose is conscious and deliberate.

More often, it is not.

The man who refuses to leave his bedroom is not calculating the effect of his refusal.

He is doing the only thing that feels possible in that moment.

Creating a boundary around the last space that still feels safe.

The woman who escalates when a request is repeated is not choosing to cause difficulty.

She is responding to what repetition has come to mean inside her chain. Pressure, loss of control, the familiar shape of a situation that has always ended badly.

The young person who goes silent and unreachable in the middle of a session is not being deliberately obstructive.

They have reached a point within the chain where withdrawal is the only regulation available.

In each case, the behaviour makes sense.

Not to the observer.

To the person living it.

And when behaviour makes sense to the person living it, correcting it from the outside without attending to what produced it is rarely effective.

There is a particular kind of behaviour that deserves careful attention in support settings.

It is behaviour that works.

When a person escalates and the source of pressure is removed, they have learned something.

When a person withdraws and the demand placed upon them disappears, they have learned something.

When a person creates enough disruption that the situation changes around them, they have learned something.

What they have learned is not always what we would choose for them to learn.

But learning has occurred.

Over time, behaviour that achieves a desired outcome becomes more likely to be repeated.

Not because the person is manipulative.

Not because they are deliberately exploiting the situation.

But because human beings, like all living things, move toward what works.

When escalation reliably produces relief, escalation becomes a strategy.

When withdrawal reliably reduces demand, withdrawal becomes a tool.

When disruption reliably shifts the environment, disruption becomes a language.

Understanding this does not mean accepting harmful behaviour without response.

It means recognising that the behaviour has a function, and that responding only to the behaviour itself, without understanding the function it serves, is unlikely to produce lasting change.

The question to ask is not only: how do we stop this behaviour?

It is: what need is this behaviour meeting, and how else might that need be addressed?

Behaviour exists on a spectrum.

At one end are behaviours that are barely perceptible.

A slight withdrawal from conversation.

A change in tone.

A reduction in eye contact.

A stillness that was not there before.

These early behavioural signals are often the most important, and the most overlooked.

They are the chain beginning to show its strain before the fragile link has given way.

A support worker who can recognise these early signals, who has developed the capacity to notice the slight shift before it becomes a significant one, has access to a window of opportunity that closes quickly. The static links in a person's chain, their history, their trauma, their long-standing patterns, set the conditions. It is the dynamic links, the environment on this particular day, the quality of sleep last night, the interaction that happened an hour ago, that tip the balance.

In that window, adjustments can be made.

To the environment.

To the approach.

To the pace of the interaction.

To the demands being placed.

Small changes, made early, can reduce the pressure within the chain before behaviour escalates to a point where both the person and those around them feel out of control.

At the other end of the spectrum are behaviours that are significant and visible.

Verbal aggression. Physical agitation. Complete shutdown. Crisis.

By the time behaviour has reached this point, the window for early intervention has already closed.

The chain has given way.

The priority now is safety, containment, and de-escalation, not explanation or correction.

Understanding where on the spectrum a person's behaviour currently sits and tracking the movement along that spectrum in real time, is one of the most practical skills a support worker can develop.

Behaviour also communicates.

Even when a person cannot find the words to describe their internal experience, and many cannot, particularly in moments of high activation, their behaviour is already speaking.

It is saying: I have reached my limit.

It is saying: something in this environment is not safe for me.

It is saying: I am not able to do what is being asked of me right now.

It is saying: I need something to change, and I do not have another way to say so.

A support worker who can hear behaviour as communication, rather than receiving it as provocation, rejection, or deliberate disruption, is positioned to respond in a fundamentally different way.

Not by agreeing with the behaviour.

Not by abandoning expectations or boundaries.

But by acknowledging what is being communicated, before addressing how it is being communicated.

That sequence matters.

Acknowledgement before correction.

Attunement before expectation.

Connection before redirection.

When these steps are reversed, when the behaviour is addressed before the communication beneath it has been heard, the chain rarely settles.

It often intensifies.

Because a person who does not feel heard will find another way to say what they need to say.

And the next attempt is rarely quieter than the last.

Reflection: Seeing Behaviour as the End, Not the Beginning

Think of a situation in which someone's behaviour surprised, frustrated, or confused you.

It may have been a client, a colleague, a family member, or someone you encountered briefly.

Rather than starting with the behaviour itself, work backwards through the chain.

What might the environment have been contributing in the lead-up to that moment?

What might the person have interpreted about the situation?

What memories or past experiences might have shaped that interpretation?

What understanding might they have arrived at about what was happening?

What emotion might that understanding have activated?

What might they have been expecting to happen next?

And then, having moved through all of those links:

Does the behaviour still seem as surprising?

This is not an exercise in excusing behaviour.

It is an exercise in understanding it.

When behaviour can be understood, when the chain that led to it becomes visible, it is no longer simply a problem to be managed.

It becomes information.

Information that can be used to intervene earlier, respond more effectively, and support the person more meaningfully.

Closing: Behaviour as the Beginning of Understanding

Behaviour is the visible end of a chain that began long before anyone watching could see it.

It is shaped by environment and interpretation.

By memory and understanding.

By the emotional states that understanding activates.

By the expectations, those emotions generate about what is coming next.

By the time behaviour appears, all of this has already occurred.

This is why responses that focus only on the behaviour itself, that treat the visible action as the starting point rather than the endpoint, so often fall short.

They are addressing the final link without attending to the chain that produced it.

Understanding behaviour through the lens of the chain does not make support work easier.

It makes it more honest.

It requires us to look further back than is always comfortable.

To consider influences that may be invisible.

To hold complexity in situations that press us toward simple explanations.

But the reward for that effort is significant.

When behaviour is understood rather than simply managed, relationships become more stable.

Interventions become more targeted.

And the people at the centre of the chain, the ones whose behaviour has been the subject of observation, assessment, and response, begin to experience something that many have not experienced enough of.

Being seen.

Not just for what they do.

For everything that led them there.

Part Two has walked the full length of the chain.

From the environment that first places pressure on the links, through the internal processes of interpretation, memory, understanding, emotion, and expectation, to the behaviour that finally becomes visible at the end.

Each link is individual.

Each chain is unique.

And the interaction between links is fluid, dynamic, and shaped by everything the person carries into each moment.

But knowing the chain exists is only the beginning.

The real question, the one that matters most for the people delivering care and support, is what to do with this knowledge.

How do you recognise the chain before it reaches its fragile point?

How do you manage your own chain while supporting someone else's?

How do teams work together in a way that strengthens rather than strains the chains of the people they support?

These are the questions that Part Three is built to answer.

CHAPTER NINE

Spotting the Chain Early

Reading Signs Before Behaviour Appears

Understanding the chain is one thing.

Seeing it in motion is another.

The preceding chapters have traced the journey from environment through to behaviour, the internal sequence that unfolds, often without words, before anything visible occurs.

That understanding is valuable.

But knowledge of the chain is most useful when it can be applied in real time.

Before the voice rises.

Before the door closes.

Before the fragile link gives way.

This chapter is about developing the capacity to read the chain while it is still forming.

To notice the early signals that pressure is building.

To recognise the moment, before it becomes a crisis, when something within the interaction needs to shift.

It is one of the most practical skills available to anyone working in a care or support role.

And like most skills of real value, it requires attention, patience, and the willingness to look at what is easy to overlook.

Early signals exist in every chain.

They are present before behaviour escalates to the point where it demands a response.

They are often subtle, easily attributed to something else, or dismissed as insignificant in the moment.

But they are there.

A slight change in posture.

A shift in eye contact, too much, or suddenly too little.

A tone that is fractionally sharper than usual.

A silence that has a different quality to it.

A response that is shorter than expected.

A body that has become still in a way that stillness does not usually mean.

None of these signals, in isolation, constitutes a crisis.

Each of them, in context, is the chain showing its strain.

The support worker who notices these signals early, who has developed what might be called a calibrated attention to the people they support, is not responding to behaviour.

They are responding to the chain before behaviour becomes necessary.

Calibrated attention is not the same as hypervigilance.

Hypervigilance is a state of chronic alertness driven by anxiety.

It exhausts the person who carries it and distorts their reading of situations, finding threat where none exists.

Calibrated attention is something quieter and more grounded.

It is built from familiarity with a person, from knowing their baseline.

Knowing what a good morning looks and sounds like for this particular individual.

Knowing how they carry themselves when they are settled.

Knowing the particular way their voice changes when something is building internally.

Knowing which environments tend to increase strain on their chain and which tend to reduce it.

This kind of knowledge does not come from assessment tools or documentation alone.

It comes from time spent alongside a person.

From the accumulated experience of many interactions, each one adding to a picture that becomes more detailed and more useful over time.

It is one of the most significant arguments for continuity of support.

When a person is supported by the same workers over time, those workers develop a baseline understanding that is genuinely protective.

They can notice when something is different before they can name what it is.

They can feel the shift in the room before the shift becomes a scene.

When workers rotate frequently, that baseline is lost.

Every interaction begins from a less informed starting point.

The early signals are harder to read because there is no foundation of familiarity to read them against.

A support worker has been working with a woman for eighteen months.

She knows her well, well enough to notice on a Thursday afternoon that something is different before a single word has been exchanged.

The woman answers the door.

The greeting is as it always is.

The words are the same.

But the worker notices something in the quality of the response.

A flatness that is not usually there.

A fraction of a second's delay before the smile that normally arrives quickly.

The worker does not immediately name what she has noticed.

She does not say: you seem off today.

She does not press for an explanation.

She simply adjusts her approach.

She slows down.

She does not move immediately into the plan for the session.

She takes a few minutes to sit, to offer tea, to allow the space between them to settle before anything is asked of it.

Later in the session, when the environment feels calmer and the woman has had time to regulate, she mentions, without prompting, that she had hard news the previous evening.

The worker's early recognition of the chain's strain did not prevent the difficulty.

But it changed the shape of the interaction around it.

The session did not escalate.

The woman did not need to use behaviour to communicate that she was not ready.

The worker saw the chain early enough to meet it before it reached the fragile point.

Reading the chain early requires attention to several domains simultaneously.

The first is the person's physical presentation.

The body communicates the state of the chain before words do.

Tension held in the jaw, the shoulders, the hands.

Shallow breathing.

Increased movement or unusual stillness.

Skin colour changes that accompany physiological arousal.

These are signals from the nervous system, visible on the surface of the body, long before behaviour escalates.

The second is the quality of communication.

Not only the content of what is said, but how it is said.

Pace, volume, tone, and the spaces between words all carry information about the state of the chain.

A person who is speaking more quickly than usual, or more slowly.

A person whose answers have become single words where they are usually sentences.

A person who is answering a different question to the one being asked.

The third is engagement with the environment.

How the person is relating to the space around them.

Whether they are orienting toward the interaction or away from it.

Whether their attention is scattered or fixed.

Whether the environment itself, its noise, its demands, its unpredictability, appears to be adding to the strain they are carrying.

The fourth is the history of this particular chain.

Every person has patterns within their chain.

Certain times of day, certain kinds of interactions, certain environmental conditions that reliably increase pressure.

A worker who knows these patterns can anticipate the conditions under which the chain is likely to be under strain and can prepare the interaction accordingly.

None of these domains provides certainty.

Together, they provide a picture.

What a worker does with that picture matters as much as the recognition itself.

Noticing that a chain is under strain is the first step.

Responding in a way that reduces rather than adds to that strain is the second.

This requires a particular kind of restraint.

When a worker notices early signs of escalating pressure, the instinct can be to address it directly.

To name it. To explain it. To problem-solve it.

But a person whose chain is already under strain is not always ready to be engaged with cognitively.

Direct questions can feel like pressure.

Naming the observation can feel like exposure.

Problem-solving can feel like being managed.

What is often more effective in the early stages is adjustment without announcement.

Slowing the pace of interaction.

Reducing the number of demands in the environment.

Offering choice where choice is possible.

Introducing familiarity and predictability.

Simply being present without agenda.

These adjustments communicate something to the nervous system that words often cannot.

They signal: this space is safe.

There is no pressure here.

You do not need to protect yourself in this moment.

That signal, received by a chain under strain, can be enough to prevent the fragile link from giving way.

There will be times when the chain cannot be caught early.

When the strain has been building outside the worker's presence.

When the pressure within the chain has reached the fragile point before anyone with the capacity to help has become involved.

In these moments, the skill is not early recognition.

It is grounded response.

Remaining calm when the environment is not calm.

Maintaining consistency when the person in front of you is anything but consistent.

Holding the boundaries of the interaction without escalating the intensity within it.

These are not small things.

They require a regulated nervous system, a sense of purpose, and crucially, a worker who understands their own chain well enough to manage it under pressure.

Which is exactly where the next chapter begins.

Reflection: Developing Your Baseline Knowledge

Choose one person you support regularly.

Without referring to documentation, consider what you actually know about their baseline.

What does a settled morning look and feel like for them?

What does their voice sound like when they are regulated?

How do they carry themselves when the chain is under minimal strain?

Now consider the early signals.

What are the first things that change when pressure begins to build within their chain?

Is it physical? Communicative? Relational?

What is the first signal you notice, before anything else shifts?

And finally, consider your response.

When you have noticed that early signal in the past, what have you done?

What has been most effective in reducing the pressure at that early stage?

What has, perhaps unintentionally, added to it?

This reflection does not need to produce conclusions.

It is an exercise in building the kind of deliberate attention that makes early recognition possible.

The more clearly you can see a person's chain in motion, the more opportunity you have to meet them before the fragile link gives way.

Closing: The Value of Seeing Early

The behaviour chain rarely announces itself.

It builds quietly, through links that are personal and often invisible, until the pressure within it becomes too great to contain.

By the time behaviour appears, the chain has already done most of its work.

The opportunity for early intervention has passed.

But before that moment, in the signals that precede it, in the shifts that are easy to miss and easier to overlook, there is a window.

A worker who can see that window, and who knows how to move within it, changes what becomes possible.

Not every escalation will be prevented.

Not every chain will be interrupted before the fragile link gives way.

But some can.

And the ones that can be caught early are the ones that
most often are, by workers who have taken the time to
know the people they support well enough to see what
is coming before it arrives.

In the next chapter, we turn the lens inward.

Because the chain being observed is not the only chain
in the room.

The worker has one too.

And understanding your own chain is not separate from
the work of supporting others.

It is at the very heart of it.

CHAPTER TEN

Your Own Chain

The Worker Inside the Situation

Every chapter in this book has looked outward.

At the client, whose environment places strain on their chain.

At the person, whose interpretation is shaped by memories they may not be able to name.

At the individual whose behaviour, when it finally appears, is the visible end of a journey that began long before anyone else could see it.

That outward focus is necessary and valuable.

But it is incomplete.

Because the support worker is not standing outside the chain they are observing.

They are standing inside it.

They bring their own environment into every interaction.

Their own interpretations.

Their own memories.

Their own understanding of what is happening and why.

Their own emotional responses.

Their own expectations about how the interaction will unfold.

The worker has a chain.

And that chain is active in every moment of every shift.

Ignoring this does not make it less true.

It simply means the chain operates without awareness.

And a chain that operates without awareness is far more likely to influence an interaction in ways the worker neither intended nor noticed.

This is not a comfortable chapter to write.
It will not always be a comfortable chapter to read.

Because it asks something of the person in the support role that is rarely asked explicitly.

Not just: can you see the chain in the person you are supporting?

But: can you see the chain in yourself?

Can you recognise the moments when your own interpretation is being shaped by something other than what is in front of you?

When your emotional response belongs as much to your history as to the present situation?

When your expectation of how this interaction will go is already directing your behaviour before the interaction has properly begun?

These are not easy questions.

They are not asked to produce shame or self-criticism.

They are asked because the answer to them is one of the most significant factors in the quality of support that becomes possible.

A worker with seven years of experience in disability support has developed a strong professional identity.

She is competent, reliable, and genuinely committed to the people she supports.

She also grew up in a household where conflict was unpredictable and often felt dangerous.

As a child, she learned to read the emotional temperature of a room before entering it.

She learned to manage her own responses carefully, to keep things calm, to absorb tension rather than contribute to it.

These skills served her then.

They serve her now, in some ways.

Her capacity to remain outwardly calm in elevated situations is considerable.

But something else has also developed alongside those skills.

When a client becomes emotionally elevated, her body responds before her training does.

There is a tightening, a heightening of alertness, a shift in her internal state that arrives before any deliberate thought.

In most situations, she manages this well enough.

But on days when she is fatigued, when her personal life is under strain, when she has moved through several hard interactions before this one, the gap between her internal response and her outward behaviour narrows.

She becomes more directive than she intends to be.

Her communication becomes slightly more controlled, slightly less warm.

She moves the interaction toward resolution more quickly than the client's chain can follow.

She is not aware that this is happening.

She experiences herself as managing the situation professionally.

The client, whose nervous system is already activated, registers something in the worker's changed quality of presence.

They cannot name it.

But they feel it.

And the chain, which might have settled with a little more time and a little less directed energy, moves instead toward its fragile point.

The worker's chain operates through the same links as everyone else's.

Environment, meaning the physical and relational context of the shift, the drive to work, the team dynamics, the handover that went badly, the news received that morning before leaving the house.

Interpretation, meaning the meaning assigned to the client's early signals, shaped by the worker's own history of how situations like this tend to unfold.

Memory, meaning the accumulated experience of previous difficult interactions, of training that did or did not prepare them, of relationships in their personal life that bear an unexamined resemblance to the dynamic in front of them.

Understanding, meaning the working conclusion the worker reaches about what is happening, who is responsible for it, and what it requires of them.

Emotion, meaning the internal response to that understanding, which may include anxiety, frustration, helplessness, protectiveness, or a complex mixture of all of these.

Expectation, meaning the anticipation formed from everything that has moved through the chain so far, of how this interaction is likely to end.

And then, at the end of all of that:

Behaviour.

The worker's tone.

Their proximity.

Their pace.

Their word choices.

Their willingness to wait.

Their capacity to remain present without directing.

Every one of these is influenced by the chain the worker is carrying.

This is not an argument for perfection.

No worker enters every interaction with a fully settled chain.

No human being does.

Fatigue, personal difficulty, professional strain, accumulated stress. These are not signs of inadequacy.

They are the conditions of a working life in a demanding sector.

The argument is not for a worker who is unaffected by their own chain.

It is for a worker who is aware of it.

Awareness changes what is possible.

A worker who knows that they are carrying strain into an interaction can make deliberate adjustments.

They can slow themselves down before entering.

They can take a breath that is not metaphorical.

They can name, even silently, what they are bringing through the door, so that it does not arrive unannounced and act without supervision.

This is not a therapeutic process.

It does not require a worker to resolve their history before they can do their job.

It simply requires a moment of honest self-awareness before the interaction begins.

Am I settled enough to be here in the way this person needs me to be?

What am I carrying today that might influence how I read this situation?

What do I need to set aside, at least for now, in order to be genuinely present?

These questions take seconds to ask.

The answers they produce can change the quality of an entire interaction.

There is a concept within therapeutic and relational practice sometimes referred to as parallel process.

It describes the way emotional dynamics in one relationship can be unconsciously replicated in another.

In support work, this can appear in a particular way.

A client who has experienced repeated abandonment may relate to their support worker in ways that subtly invite abandonment, testing limits, creating distance, behaving in ways that make continued support feel unsustainable.

A worker who has their own unexamined experiences of rejection may find themselves responding to this dynamic in ways that confirm, rather than interrupt, the client's expectation.

Not because either person has consciously chosen this outcome.

But because two chains, carrying complementary wounds, have met in the space between them and enacted a familiar pattern.

This is not inevitable.

But it is common enough to deserve attention.

When a worker finds themselves repeatedly frustrated by a particular client in ways they cannot fully explain that frustration is worth examining.

When a worker notices that certain interactions consistently activate a response that feels larger than the situation warrants, that activation is worth slowing down and looking at.

Not as a failing.

As information.

Information about where the worker's own chain carries vulnerability.

And, with the right support, information that can become the basis for growth.

Supervision, debriefing, and peer support are not optional extras in this work.

They are structural necessities.

A support worker who has no regular space to reflect on the interactions they are having, to process the emotional residue those interactions leave, and to examine their own chain with the support of another person, is a worker whose chain will gradually accumulate strain with no mechanism for release.

Over time, this strain does not disappear.

It finds its way into interactions.

Into slightly shortened patience.

Into responses that are more reactive than considered.

Into a growing distance between the worker and the genuine relational presence that effective support requires.

This is not a moral failing.

It is physics.

Pressure that has nowhere to go does not simply stop existing.

It moves somewhere else.

Organisations that take the behaviour chain seriously must therefore take seriously the chains of the people doing the work.

Supervision is not a luxury.

Debriefing after difficult incidents is not optional.

The emotional wellbeing of support workers is not separate from the quality of support delivered.

It is the foundation of it.

Reflection: Examining Your Own Chain

Set aside the people you support for a moment.

Consider your own chain.

Think of a recent shift, or a specific interaction, which left you feeling unsettled, frustrated, depleted, or reactive in a way that surprised you.

Work through the links.

What was the environment you brought into that interaction, not just the physical environment of the workplace, but the internal environment you arrived with?

What did you interpret about the situation?

Was that interpretation shaped by something beyond what was directly in front of you?

What memories or past experiences might have contributed to the way you read the moment?

What did you understand was happening, and how much of that understanding was about the present situation, and how much was about something older?

What emotion was activated?

Where did you feel it?

What were you expecting would happen?

And did that expectation change how you behaved before the anticipated outcome had even arrived?

There are no right answers here.

There is only honest looking.

The worker who can examine their own chain with this kind of honesty is not a perfect worker.

They are a self-aware one.

And self-awareness, in this work, is one of the most protective factors available, for the people being supported and for the worker themselves.

Closing: The Worker as Part of the System

Support work is relational work.

It cannot be delivered from a position of complete neutrality, because no such position exists.

The worker is always inside the interaction.

Always bringing something.

Always, whether they know it or not, influencing the chain of the person they are supporting through the state of their own.

This is not a burden.

It is a responsibility.

And it is also an opportunity.

A worker whose chain is relatively settled, who enters an interaction with presence and a regulated nervous system, communicates something to the person they are supporting that no words can replicate.

Safety.

Predictability.

The sense that this space can be trusted.

For people, whose chains have been shaped by environments that offered very little safety, very little predictability, and very little reason to trust, these are not small things at all.

The worker's chain matters.

Not as a limitation to be apologised for.

As a resource to be cultivated.

In the next chapter, we move from the individual worker to the team.

Because when multiple workers are supporting the same person, multiple chains are in play.

And what happens when those chains are inconsistent is one of the most significant and underexamined sources of strain in support settings.

CHAPTER ELEVEN

Team Consistency

When Chains Collide

A person is not supported by a single worker.

In most disability and community support settings, a person may interact with several different workers across the course of a week.

Different faces at the door.

Different communication styles.

Different interpretations of what the support plan requires.

Different levels of comfort with boundaries, flexibility, and relational warmth.

Each of these workers brings their own chain into every interaction.

Their own histories, interpretations, emotional responses, and expectations.

And the person at the centre of all of this, the one whose chain is already shaped by everything they carry, must navigate not one chain meeting theirs, but many.

When those many chains are inconsistent with each other, the person does not experience a support team.

They experience a series of unpredictable encounters, each one requiring them to recalibrate, to reassess safety, to re-establish what the rules of this particular interaction are going to be.

That recalibration is exhausting.

And exhaustion adds strain to the chain.

Consider what consistency actually means within the behaviour chain.

It does not mean that every worker must have the same personality.

It does not mean that warmth, humour, or individual relational style must be suppressed in favour of a uniform approach.

It means that the fundamental conditions of the support relationship, the expectations, the boundaries, the responses to particular behaviours, the way requests are made and declined, are similar enough across the team that the person being supported can develop a reliable understanding of what to expect.

When this understanding is available, the expectation link in the chain is stabilised.

The person does not need to test each new interaction to establish its parameters.

They do not need to escalate in order to discover where the limits are.

They do not need to use behaviour as a mapping tool for a landscape that keeps shifting beneath them.

They already know what to expect.

And knowing what to expect is, for many people whose chains have been shaped by unpredictability and inconsistency, one of the most regulating experiences available.

A man in his late twenties is supported by a team of six workers across a seven-day roster.

Four of the workers have been with the service for some time.

They know him well. They have developed a shared understanding of his chain, including the conditions under which pressure builds, the early signals that strain is present, and the approaches that tend to settle the interaction and the ones that tend to escalate it.

Two workers joined the team recently.

They are capable and committed, but they have not yet developed the baseline familiarity that the longer-serving workers carry.

They work from the support plan, which is detailed and professionally written, but which cannot fully capture the texture of what has been learned through months of interaction.

On the days supported by the experienced workers, the man's chain tends to remain settled.

Transitions are managed smoothly. Expectations are clear. The environment feels predictable.

On the days supported by the newer workers, something different sometimes occurs.

Not always.

Not dramatically.

But often enough to be noticed.

A request is phrased in a way that feels different to him, even if the content is identical.

A limit is held less firmly, or held more rigidly, than he has come to expect.

A signal that the experienced workers would recognise and respond to passes without acknowledgment.

His chain registers these differences.

Interpretation is activated.

Familiar questions form: is this safe? What are the rules today? Can I trust what is being offered?

The strain within the chain increases.

Not because the newer workers are doing anything wrong.

But because the conditions they are creating, through no fault of their own, are different enough from what he knows to activate the parts of his chain that respond to uncertainty.

The solution here is not to expect new workers to be immediately as effective as experienced ones.

That expectation is neither fair nor realistic.

The solution is a team that treats consistency as a shared responsibility.

This begins with communication.

Handovers that go beyond logistics, which include not only what happened during the shift but how the person seemed, what signals were present, and what approaches were effective and what were not.

Team meetings that create space not only for administrative discussion but for the kind of relational reflection that builds shared understanding.

Supervision structures that include conversation about how the team as a whole is responding to a particular person, not only how individual workers are performing.

Documentation that captures not just what a person needs but why, that includes enough context about the behaviour chain that a worker reading it for the first time can begin to understand the person they are about to support, not only the tasks they are about to perform.

Inconsistency in a team does not always arise from inexperience.

It can arise from disagreement.

Workers within a team often disagree about how a person should be supported.

One worker believes that a particular behaviour should be consistently redirected.

Another believes that flexibility in certain moments is more therapeutic than firmness.

One worker allows an exception that another would not.

One worker's interpretation of what the support plan requires differs meaningfully from a colleague.

When these differences are not surfaced and discussed, they do not disappear.

They play out in the daily interactions between workers and the people they support.

And the person at the centre of the team experiences the result.

Not as a theoretical disagreement between workers.

As inconsistency in the environment, they depend on.

For a person whose chain already carries vulnerability around unpredictability, whose early experiences taught them that the rules can change without warning, that safety can be withdrawn, that what is allowed today may not be allowed tomorrow, this inconsistency is not merely inconvenient.

It is activating.

It reaches directly into the interpretation and expectation links of the chain and confirms what those links have always feared.

The ground is not reliable here.

It never is.

Team consistency is also tested in moments of escalation.

When a person's behaviour reaches its most visible and most challenging point, the team's response matters enormously.

If one worker's response is calm and containing while another's reactive and directive, the person receives conflicting information about what the escalation means and what it will produce.

If the team's approach changes depending on who is rostered, if certain workers are known to yield under pressure while others hold firm, the person's expectation link learns to calibrate its behaviour to the worker in the room.

This is not manipulation in any deliberate sense.

It is the behaviour chain doing what it is designed to do.

Learning the landscape.

Adapting to what works.

When the landscape is inconsistent, the learning it produces is inconsistent.

And behaviours that might have settled with a stable and unified team response can instead become entrenched, because the inconsistency within the team keeps the reinforcement of those behaviours alive.

There is a particular dynamic that deserves specific attention.

It occurs when one worker within a team becomes, over time, the person who manages the most difficult interactions.

Perhaps they have a natural capacity for de-escalation.

Perhaps the person responds to them in a way they do not respond to others.

Perhaps they have simply accumulated the most experience with this individual's chain.

Over time, the team may begin, informally and without explicit decision, to route difficult situations toward this worker.

They become the person who is called when things escalate.
The one who can settle what others cannot.

This dynamic, while understandable, creates several problems.

It removes the incentive for the rest of the team to develop their own capacity to manage difficulty.

It places unsustainable pressure on the worker at the centre of it.

And it creates a dependency within the person's chain that becomes its own vulnerability. When that worker is absent, the person has been inadvertently taught that safety is located in one individual rather than in the team as a whole.

Team consistency means distributing not only the routine tasks of support, but the relational and regulatory demands of it.

Every worker on the team should be developing their capacity to hold the chain with care.

Not equally, because different workers will always have different strengths.

But sufficiently that the team as a whole represents a stable and containing environment, rather than a collection of individuals with one reliable anchor.

Reflection: Examining Consistency Within Your Team

Think about the team you currently work within, or a team you have been part of in the past.

Consider the person or people being supported.

How consistent is the environment that team creates across different workers and different shifts?

Are there workers whose approach differs significantly from the team's shared understanding?

Are those differences discussed openly, or do they operate beneath the surface?

Are there particular workers who consistently manage difficulty more effectively than others?

And if so, is that capacity being shared and developed across the team, or is it concentrated in one or two individuals?

When the team disagrees about how a situation should be handled, where does that disagreement go?

Is there a forum for it to be examined and resolved?

Or does it remain unspoken and play out instead in the daily interactions with the people being supported?

These questions are not about assigning fault.

They are about recognising that a team, like an individual, has its own chain.

A collective set of influences, dynamics, and patterns that shape the environment experienced by the people at the centre of the support relationship.

When that collective chain is examined with honesty and care, it becomes possible to strengthen it.

Closing: The Team as a Containing Environment

The behaviour chain is individual.

But it does not exist in isolation.

Every person's chain is embedded in an environment.

And for many of the people accessing disability and community support, that environment includes a team of workers whose collective presence either stabilises or strains the chain on a daily basis.

A consistent team is not one without difference.

It is one where the differences are understood, discussed, and held within a shared framework of purpose and approach.

When a team achieves this, when the person being supported can move from one worker to the next and find, beneath the individual differences, a recognisable and reliable set of conditions, something significant becomes possible.

The chain begins to trust the environment.

The expectation link begins to anticipate safety rather than unpredictability.

The energy that was previously spent recalibrating to each new interaction becomes available for something else.

For growth.

For connection.

For the kind of engagement with life that good support is ultimately intended to make possible.

In the next chapter, we turn to the practical question that sits at the heart of Part Three.

When the chain reaches its fragile point, when escalation has occurred or is clearly approaching, what does effective intervention actually look like?

What works, what does not, and why.

CHAPTER TWELVE

Intervening in the Chain

Practical Tools for De-escalation

Everything in this book has been building toward a practical question.

When the chain is under strain, when pressure is building, when the fragile link is approaching, or when it has already given way, what do you actually do?

Not in theory.

In the room.

In the moment.

With a person whose chain has reached a point that demands a response.

This chapter is an attempt to answer that question as honestly and practically as possible.

Not with a formula.

Not with a sequence of steps that will work in every situation regardless of context.

But with a set of principles, grounded in the behaviour chain, that can guide the quality of a response when the pressure is real and the window for effective intervention is narrow.

The first and most important principle is this.

You cannot intervene effectively in someone else's chain while your own is dysregulated.

This has been said already, in an earlier chapter, and it is said again here because it is the foundation on which everything else rests.

Before any technique, any strategy, any carefully chosen word or deliberate adjustment to the environment, the worker's own internal state is the primary tool.

A regulated nervous system is contagious.

So is a dysregulated one.

When a worker enters an elevated situation carrying their own activation, anxiety held in the shoulders, urgency in the pace of movement, tightness in the voice, the person they are trying to support receives that signal before any words are spoken.

The nervous system does not wait for language.

It reads the room.

And a room in which the person attempting to help is also activated does not feel safe.

It feels like two chains in difficulty, rather than one chain being met by something steadier.

So, the first intervention is always internal.

Breath.

Pace.

The deliberate choice to slow the body before attempting to settle the environment.

This takes seconds.

It changes everything.

The second principle is to meet the emotion before addressing the behaviour.

When a person's chain has reached its fragile point, their nervous system is activated.

The parts of the brain most involved in reasoning, in weighing options, in responding to explanation, these are significantly less available than they would be in a calmer state.

Attempting to reason with a dysregulated person is not ineffective because they are being deliberately difficult.

It is ineffective because the neurobiology of dysregulation makes reasoning genuinely harder to access.

What is available, even in high states of activation, is the capacity to feel heard.

Not agreed with.

Not validated in every conclusion they have reached.

Simply heard.

When a worker communicates, through tone, through presence, through the quality of their attention, that they are not here to argue, not here to correct, not here to manage, but to understand, something shifts.

Not every intervention lands.

A support worker has read the signs correctly. She has noticed the early signals, regulated her own chain, and approached the situation with genuine calm. She reduces her demands, lowers her voice, and creates space for the person to settle.

But the escalation continues.

She tries again. She offers choices. She names what she is observing without judgment. She does everything the framework would suggest.

And still the chain does not settle.

Afterward, she sits with her team leader and works through what happened. Together they look at the links.

The environment had been strained for days, not hours. A visiting family member had been present throughout the week, and the dynamic between them carried its own history. The support worker had read the signals of the present moment accurately but had not known about the accumulated pressure that had been building long before her shift began.

She had intervened at the right moment. She had simply not had access to the full chain.

This is not a failure of skill or judgment. It is a reminder that the behaviour chain belongs to the person carrying it. A worker can create the conditions for the chain to settle. They cannot force it to.

What the framework offers in these moments is not a guarantee of resolution. It is a way of understanding what happened without defaulting to blame, whether of the person who escalated, or of the worker who tried to help.

The question is not what went wrong.

It is what the chain was carrying that the intervention could not reach.

And what does that tell us about what this person needs next.

Not always dramatically.

Not always immediately.

But the shift is real.

The nervous system, receiving the signal that it is not under threat from the person in the room, begins to have less work to do.

Activation begins to reduce.

The gap between feeling and behaviour begins, gradually, to widen.

This is co-regulation.

And it is the most powerful intervention available.

What does meeting the emotion actually look like in practice?

It looks like a tone of voice that does not rise to meet the distress.

Calm, even, unhurried. Not flat or disconnected, but grounded.

It looks like language that acknowledges without inflaming.

Not: you need to calm down.

Not: there is no reason to react like this.

But: I can see this is really difficult right now.

Or simply: I am here. I am not going anywhere.

It looks like a body that is open rather than braced.

Facing the person without crowding them.

At a level, where possible, rather than standing over.

Hands visible. Posture unhurried.

It looks like silence used well.

The willingness to be present without filling every moment with words.

To allow the space between words to do some of the work.

And it looks like curiosity rather than assessment.

Not watching the person to determine their risk level.

Being with the person to understand their experience.

These are not techniques to be performed.

They are qualities to be embodied.

The difference is felt by the person receiving them.

The third principle is to reduce demand without abandoning expectation.

When a person's chain is under significant strain, the demands within the environment need to be temporarily reduced.

Not permanently.

Not as a reward for the escalation.

But as a practical recognition that a chain under pressure cannot meet the same demands as a chain at rest.

This might mean pausing the planned activity.

Reducing the number of people in the immediate environment.

Removing a sensory pressure, whether noise, lighting, or proximity, which is adding to the strain.

Offering choice where choice can be offered.

Stepping back physically to create space.

None of this means that expectations disappear.

It means that the timing of expectations is adjusted to the actual state of the chain.

There is an important distinction here that is worth naming clearly.

Reducing demand in response to escalating behaviour, with the intention of settling the chain before returning to the expectation, is sound practice.

Removing expectations entirely and permanently in response to behaviour is a different thing.

It confirms, within the person's chain, that escalation is an effective strategy for changing the environment.

And as explored in an earlier chapter, behaviour that achieves a desired outcome becomes more likely to be repeated.

The goal is not to make difficulty disappear by eliminating what caused it.

The goal is to reduce the pressure enough that the chain can settle, and then, when the person is regulated enough to engage, to return to the expectation with the same consistency that was present before the escalation occurred.

The fourth principle is to use the environment deliberately.

The environment is the first link in the chain.

It can be a source of strain.

It can also be a source of support.

In moments of escalation, the physical environment can be adjusted to reduce activation.

Moving to a quieter space.

Reducing visual clutter or stimulation.

Adjusting lighting where possible.

Introducing something familiar, an object, a routine, a sensory anchor, which is associated with safety within the person's chain.

These adjustments are not always possible.

But when they are, they work directly on the first link in the chain, reducing the input that is feeding the internal pressure.

The relational environment matters equally.

Removing additional workers from the immediate space if their presence is adding to the intensity of the situation.

Ensuring that the person is not surrounded by observers whose attention itself becomes a source of activation.

Creating a sense of containment, not physical containment, but the relational sense that this space is bounded, that the situation is manageable, that there are people present who know what to do and are not frightened by what is happening.

That last quality, the worker's lack of fear, communicates more than perhaps anything else.

A worker who is genuinely unafraid, who is stable and present in the middle of difficulty, communicates to the person in the chain that this moment is survivable.

That it will not last forever.

That something steady exists in the midst of it.

The fifth principle is to know when to step back.

There are moments in which continued engagement from a particular worker is not reducing the pressure in the chain.

It is adding to it.

Perhaps the worker has become part of the trigger.

Perhaps their presence is activating something within the person's chain that a different face would not.

Perhaps the dynamic between them has, in this particular moment, passed the point where forward movement is possible.

Knowing when to step back, and doing so without signalling defeat, rejection, or escalation, is a skill.

It requires the worker to set aside any sense that stepping back represents personal failure.

It does not.

It requires the ability to hand the interaction to a colleague in a way that maintains the consistency of the team's approach, so that the change in person does not become an additional source of instability.

And it requires the honest self-awareness to recognise when continuing to engage is about the worker's own need for resolution rather than the person's need for support.

Stepping back, when done well, can itself be de-escalating.

The change in dynamic, the introduction of a different relational presence, the removal of an interaction that has become entangled, these can allow the person's chain to reset in ways that continued engagement could not achieve.

After escalation has settled, after the chain has found its way back from the fragile point, there is work still to be done.

Not immediately.

Not while the nervous system is still returning to baseline.

But when the person is regulated, when the environment has settled, when enough time has passed that the interaction can be revisited without reactivation, there is value in what might simply be called returning.

Returning to connection.

A brief acknowledgement that something difficult happened, without dwelling in it.

A reaffirmation of the relationship that was present before the escalation and remains present after it.

And, where appropriate and when the person has the capacity for it, a gentle curiosity about what was happening within the chain.

Not as an inquest.

Not as a lesson.

But as an invitation.

What was going on for you earlier?

Is there anything that would have helped?

Is there something we can do differently next time?

These conversations, held carefully and without pressure, can become some of the most valuable interactions in a support relationship.

They build insight within the person about their own chain.

They communicate that the worker's interest in them does not diminish when things are difficult.

And they lay the groundwork for a different outcome the next time pressure builds.

Reflection: Reviewing a Difficult Interaction

Think of a recent interaction in which a person's chain reached a point of visible escalation.

Work through the following questions, not to find fault, but to find understanding.

At what point did you first notice the chain was under strain?

What signals were present that, looking back, indicated pressure was building?

What was your own internal state at the moment you recognised the escalation?

Were you regulated enough to respond from a settled place, or were you carrying strain of your own?

What did you do first?

And looking back, did that response meet the emotion, or did it address the behaviour before the emotion had been acknowledged?

What in the environment was adding to the pressure?

Was anything adjusted? Could anything have been adjusted earlier?

How did the interaction end?

And was there a moment of return, a reconnection after the difficulty had passed?

This reflection is not about perfecting what has already happened.

It is about building the kind of honest examination of practice that makes the next difficult interaction a little more navigable than the last.

Closing: Intervention as Relationship

De-escalation is not a set of techniques applied to a problem.

It is a relational act performed by one human being for another.

The tools in this chapter, the regulated presence, the validation of emotion, the adjusted demand, the deliberate use of environment, the willingness to step back and to return, these are only effective when they are offered genuinely.

When the worker is truly present.

When the curiosity about the person's experience is real.

When the stability being offered is not a performance of calm but an actual internal state.

These qualities cannot be manufactured in the moment.

They are built over time, through self-awareness, through supervision, through the accumulated experience of interactions that did not go well and were examined honestly afterward.

Intervention in the behaviour chain is, ultimately, the work of one chain reaching toward another with steadiness and care.

Not to fix.

Not to correct.

But to be present in a way that allows the other chain to find its way back from the fragile point.

That is what good support looks like in its hardest moments.

And it is what the people at the centre of these chains deserve to receive.

In the final chapter of this book, we step back from the individual interaction and look at the broader question.

What does it look like when an entire organisation understands the behaviour chain?

What changes?

What becomes possible?

And what is required of the people who lead these organisations to make that vision real?

CHAPTER THIRTEEN

Building Chain-Aware Organisations

Culture, Supervision, and Systemic Change

Everything explored in this book has begun with the individual.

The individual whose chain is shaped by environment, interpretation, memory, understanding, emotion, and expectation.

The individual worker whose own chain is active in every interaction they deliver.

The individual team whose collective consistency either stabilises or strains the chains of the people they support.

But individuals exist within systems.

And systems either support the principles explored in this book, or they quietly undermine them, regardless of how skilled, committed, or self-aware the individuals within those systems might be.

This is the chapter that addresses the system.

It is written for the people who lead organisations, manage teams, design policies, and shape the cultures within which support work takes place.

But it is also written for the frontline worker who has ever felt that the organisation they work within was making their job harder than it needed to be, and who has wondered why the gap between what good support looks like in theory and what it looks like in practice seems so difficult to close.

That gap is rarely the result of individual failure.

It is almost always the result of a system that has not been designed with the behaviour chain in mind.

An organisation has a chain.

This is not a metaphor.

Just as an individual moves through environment, interpretation, memory, understanding, emotion, and expectation before behaviour becomes visible, an organisation moves through its own version of these links.

The environment the organisation creates, the physical spaces, the rostering structures, the communication systems, the policies that govern daily practice, places pressure on or removes pressure from the chains of everyone within it.

The way the organisation interprets difficulty, whether behavioural incidents are understood as individual failures, as systemic signals, or as information about the state of the chains involved, shapes how the organisation responds.

The memory the organisation carries, its history of critical incidents, of staff turnover, of previous approaches that did or did not work, influences the understanding it reaches about what is happening and what is required.

The emotions the organisation activates in its workers, through the quality of supervision, the adequacy of support, the sense of being valued or expendable, determine the emotional state that workers carry into every interaction they deliver.

And the expectations the organisation holds, about what good support looks like, about what behaviour management requires, about what is acceptable and what is not, shape the behaviour of everyone within the system.

When an organisation's chain is under strain, the people at the end of it, the clients, residents, and community members receiving support, feel it.

Not because the workers are failing them.

Because the system is failing the workers.

A chain-aware organisation begins with how it understands behaviour.

Not just the behaviour of the people it supports.

The behaviour of everyone within the system.

When a support worker responds reactively to a client's escalation, a chain-aware organisation does not ask only: what did this worker do wrong?

It asks: what was happening within this worker's chain at the time? What in the system contributed to that?

What support was or was not available? What could be changed to produce a different outcome next time?

When a team becomes inconsistent in its approach to a particular person, a chain-aware organisation does not ask only: which workers are not following the plan?

It asks: what in the team's dynamic has created this inconsistency? Are there unresolved disagreements? Is supervision adequate? Does the team have the shared understanding it needs to work together effectively?

When a person's behaviour escalates repeatedly despite multiple interventions, a chain-aware organisation does not ask only: what further restrictions or consequences are required?

It asks: what links in this person's chain are under consistent strain? What in the environment we are creating is contributing to that strain? What have we not yet understood about what this person needs?

This shift in questioning, from individual blame to systemic understanding, is the foundation of a chain-aware culture.

It does not mean that individual accountability disappears.

It means that accountability is located accurately, at the level of the system as well as the individual, and with genuine curiosity about what produced the outcome rather than only who is responsible for it.

Supervision is the structural heartbeat of a chain-aware organisation.

Not supervision as administrative oversight.

Not supervision as performance monitoring.

Supervision as a genuine space for the worker's chain to be examined, supported, and strengthened.

A supervision session in a chain-aware organisation might include:

A review of recent interactions, not to assess whether the worker followed protocol, but to explore what was happening within the chains involved, including the worker's own.

An examination of any moments of difficulty, with curiosity rather than judgment, looking for what the interaction revealed about the chains at play and what might be done differently.

Attention to the worker's own wellbeing, because a worker whose chain is consistently under strain without adequate support will eventually reach their own fragile point, and the consequences of that reaching extend to everyone they support.

Space for the worker to name what they are finding difficult, the clients whose chains are hardest to hold, the team dynamics that are creating friction, the aspects of the role that are depleting rather than sustaining.

And a consistent return to the purpose of the work, to the question of what the people at the centre of the support relationship actually need, and whether the current approach is genuinely serving that need.

Supervision structured in this way is not a luxury.

It is the mechanism through which chain awareness is maintained across an entire organisation over time.

When supervision is reduced, delegated to paperwork, or experienced by workers as something done to them rather than for them, the chains within the organisation accumulate strain with no mechanism for release.

The consequences appear eventually.

In staff turnover.

In burnout.

In the quiet erosion of the relational quality that makes support work meaningful and effective.

Training in a chain-aware organisation is not a one-time event.

It is an ongoing conversation.

The Behaviour Chain Principle is not a framework that can be absorbed in a half-day induction and then applied reliably under pressure.

It requires repeated engagement, reflection, and the opportunity to examine real situations through its lens over time.

A chain-aware organisation builds this into its rhythms.

Regular team discussions that use the chain as a shared language for understanding what is happening with particular clients.

Case reflection processes that examine difficult interactions through the links of the chain rather than simply documenting what occurred.

Peer learning structures that allow workers to share what they have observed and learned with each other in a way that builds collective chain awareness across the team.

When the behaviour chain becomes the shared language of an organisation, when workers, team leaders, and managers all use the same framework to understand and discuss behaviour, something significant shifts.

Conversations become more precise.

Misunderstandings about the meaning of behaviour become less frequent.

Responses to difficulty become more coordinated.

And the people being supported experience the result, a more consistent, more attuned, more genuinely understanding environment around them.

A chain-aware organisation takes its physical environments seriously.

The spaces in which support is delivered are not neutral.

They are the first link in every chain of every person who moves through them.

Environments that are noisy, unpredictable, overcrowded, or poorly resourced place strain on chains before any interaction has begun.

Environments that are calm, predictable, appropriately stimulating, and designed with the sensory and regulatory needs of the people using them in mind reduce strain before it needs to be managed.

This is not always within the organisation's control.

Community settings, client homes, and shared facilities come with constraints that cannot always be overcome.

But where design choices can be made, in group accommodation, in day programs, in support offices, in the structures of rosters and routines, a chain-aware organisation makes them with the behaviour chain explicitly in mind.

Not as an afterthought.

As a design principle.

Leadership in a chain-aware organisation models what it asks of others.

This deserves direct statement.

An organisation cannot ask its workers to develop self-awareness about their own chains while its leaders remain unexamined.

It cannot ask frontline staff to regulate under pressure while its managers communicate urgency, anxiety, and reactive energy into the system.

It cannot ask teams to hold consistency while the organisation itself shifts its expectations, its priorities, and its tolerance for difficulty depending on who is asking and how loudly.

Leaders have chains.

Those chains are felt throughout the organisations they lead.

A leader who responds to critical incidents with blame rather than curiosity activates the defensive and self-protective responses of every worker in the system.

A leader who communicates that workers are expendable, that their wellbeing is secondary to compliance and output, creates an organisational environment in which chain-aware practice is simply not sustainable.

Conversely, a leader who models genuine curiosity about behaviour, who asks what produced this rather than who is to blame for it, creates a culture in which the same question becomes safe for everyone to ask.

A leader who takes the chains of their workers seriously, who ensures adequate supervision, who makes debriefing a genuine rather than a performative process, who communicates that the emotional demands of this work are real and worthy of attention, creates an organisation whose chains are, on balance, more stable than they would otherwise be.

This is not soft management.

It is the most practical thing a leader in this sector can do.

The measure of a chain-aware organisation is not the absence of behavioural incidents.

Chains will always reach their fragile points.

That is the nature of human beings living under pressure in a world that is rarely perfectly calibrated to their needs.

The measure is what the organisation does when those moments occur.

Whether it responds with curiosity or blame.

Whether it supports the workers involved or leaves them to carry the weight alone.

Whether it uses the incident as an opportunity to understand the chain more deeply, or files it away as a deviation from the expected.

Whether, in the weeks and months that follow, anything actually changes.

A chain-aware organisation learns.

Not despite its hard moments.

From them.

It treats every incident as information.

Every moment of escalation as a signal worth decoding.

Every pattern of behaviour, in clients, in workers, in teams, as data about the state of the chains within the system.

And it uses that information, consistently and with genuine commitment, to build an environment in which the chains of the people it exists to serve are less likely to reach their fragile point.

Not because difficulty has gone.

Because the system has become good enough at recognising and responding to the chain that it can meet difficulty before it becomes crisis, and support recovery after crisis with the consistency and care that makes a genuine difference.

Reflection: Examining Your Organisation's Chain

Consider the organisation you currently work within, or one you have been part of.

Think about the environment it creates for the workers within it.

Does that environment add to or reduce the strain on the chains of the people delivering support?

Consider how the organisation understands behaviour, both the behaviour of clients and the behaviour of staff.

Is the first question asked one of blame, or one of curiosity?

Think about the supervision structures available.

Do they genuinely support the worker's chain, or are they primarily administrative?

Consider how the organisation responds to difficulty.

Does it learn from critical incidents, or does it manage them?

And finally, think about the leadership.

Does it model what it asks of others?

Does it communicate, through its actions as well as its stated values, that the chains of the people doing this work genuinely matter?

These questions are not asked to produce cynicism.

They are asked to support the kind of honest organisational self-examination that makes change possible.

Because organisations, like individuals, can only develop awareness of their chain if someone is willing to look at it honestly.

Closing: What Becomes Possible

A chain-aware organisation is not a perfect one.

It is one that has committed to understanding behaviour, all behaviour at every level of the system, as meaningful, connected, and shaped by influences that can be examined and addressed.

It is one that has built the structures, the cultures, and the leadership practices that make chain-aware support not just theoretically possible but practically sustainable.

And it is one that holds, at the centre of everything it does, a clear and honest answer to the question of why any of this matters.

It matters because the people at the centre of the chain deserve it.

The people whose environments have shaped them in ways they did not choose.

Whose interpretations carry the weight of experiences they did not ask for.

Whose memories hold things that have made trusting the world genuinely difficult.

Whose understanding of what is happening is filtered through a history of being misread, managed, and misjudged.

Whose emotions others called problems when they were signals.

Whose expectations of support formed in environments that offered very little to expect.

These people deserve to be seen.

Truly seen.

Not as the behaviour at the end of the chain.

But as the full human being whose chain it is.

That is what a chain-aware organisation makes possible.

Not in every moment.

Not without effort, difficulty, and setback.

But consistently enough, and with enough genuine care, that the people at the centre of the chain begin to experience something that changes the links within it.

The slow, accumulating experience of being understood.

And that experience, over time, is one of the most powerful forces for change available.

In the conclusion that follows, we return to where this book began.

With a single moment.

A comment made.

A response that surprised.

A behaviour that appeared suddenly and left everyone wondering what had just happened.

And now, having walked the full length of the chain, we look at that moment again.

With different eyes.

CONCLUSION

The Chain Never Breaks

It Evolves

Come back to the beginning.

A comment is made.

A look is exchanged.

A message is received.

And something shifts.

A voice rises that was not raised a moment ago.

A person withdraws from a conversation they were present in a second before.

A behaviour appears, seemingly from nowhere, and leaves everyone around it wondering what just happened.

This is where the book began.

With that moment of apparent suddenness.

That sense of a reaction arriving without warning, disproportionate to the situation, difficult to explain.

You have now walked the full length of the chain that produces that moment.

You have seen the environment that placed the first pressure on the links.

You have followed the interpretation that transformed an external event into something personal and charged.

You have watched memory carry the weight of experiences that were never fully resolved into a present moment that resembled them.

You have traced the understanding that formed, not always accurately, not always consciously, about what was happening and what it meant.

You have felt the emotion that understanding activated, and the way that emotion reached forward into anticipation.

You have seen the expectation that formed about what was coming next, and how that expectation shaped behaviour before the anticipated event had even arrived.

And then, at the end of all of that, you have seen the behaviour.

The visible, final link.

The moment that looks sudden but is not.

The reaction that appears from nowhere but has been forming, quietly and inevitably, through every link that preceded it.

You cannot unsee this.

That is the point.

Once the chain becomes visible, behaviour stops being a mystery.

It does not stop being difficult.

It does not stop being challenging to sit with, to respond to, or to manage in the moment when the pressure is real and the options feel limited.

But it stops being inexplicable.

And something important lives in that shift from inexplicable to understandable.

Empathy becomes possible where judgment previously lived.

Curiosity becomes possible where frustration previously lived.

A different kind of response becomes possible, one that addresses not only the behaviour at the end of the chain, but the pressures within the chain that produced it.

This is what the Behaviour Chain Principle offers.

Not a solution to every difficult situation.

Not a guarantee that escalation can always be prevented or that every fragile link can be strengthened before it gives way.

But a framework for seeing behaviour as connected rather than random.

As meaningful rather than arbitrary.

As the visible expression of an internal experience that deserves to be understood.

The chain never fully breaks.

Even in the hardest moments, when behaviour has escalated to its most visible and most challenging point, the chain is still there.

Still connected.

Still carrying information about what the person needs and what the environment has failed to provide.

After the moment passes, the chain begins to rebuild.

New experiences are added to it.

New interactions shape its links.

New environments either add to its strain or begin, gradually, to reduce it.

This is the source of hope within the Behaviour Chain Principle.

A chain is not fixed.

It is not a life sentence written in the links of a person's history.

It is a living system.

One that responds to experience.

One that can, with the right conditions, develop new capacity, for regulation, for trust, for the kind of engagement with the world that may have felt impossible when the chain was under its greatest strain.

Those conditions do not arrive by accident.

They are created.

By support workers who show up consistently and see the person before they see the behaviour.

By teams who hold a shared understanding with enough care to offer genuine predictability.

By organisations who take the chains of the people they serve seriously enough to build systems worthy of that seriousness.

By leaders who model what they ask of others and hold curiosity where blame would be easier.

The chain evolves in the presence of these things.

Slowly, often.

Non-linearly, always.

With setbacks that can feel like the whole chain unravelling, even when it is not.

But it evolves.

And that evolution, witnessed over time by the people who stay alongside it with genuine commitment, is one of the most remarkable things that support work makes possible.

A final thought for the person reading this in a support role.

The work you do is not administrative.

It is not procedural.

It is not adequately captured by compliance frameworks, incident reports, or support plans, however well written those documents might be.

It is relational work.

Human work.

The work of one chain meeting another, day after day, with enough steadiness and enough genuine care to make a difference that cannot always be measured but is always felt.

You will not always get it right.

Your own chain will sometimes be under strain in moments that require more of you than you have available that day.

You will occasionally say the wrong thing, misread a signal, respond when stepping back would have served better.

This does not make you inadequate.

It makes you human.

Which is exactly what the person across from you needs you to be.

Not perfect.

Present.

Not unaffected.

Aware.

The Behaviour Chain Principle does not ask you to be more than human.

It asks you to be more human, more curious, more self-aware, more attuned to the experience of the person in front of you and to the experience of yourself in the interaction.

That is enough.

In fact, offered consistently and with genuine intention, it is more than enough.

It is the thing that changes chains.

APPENDIX

Quick Reference

The Behaviour Chain Principle

The Chain

ENVIRONMENT → INTERPRETATION → MEMORY → UNDERSTANDING → EMOTION → EXPECTATION → BEHAVIOUR

Each link is shaped by the individual.

No two chains are identical.

Behaviour is always the final link, never the first.

The Links at a Glance

Environment

The physical, sensory, and relational setting in which the person exists.

Includes noise, routine, predictability, the presence and behaviour of others, and the demands of the immediate context.

Key question: What in this environment is adding pressure to the chain?

Interpretation

The meaning assigned to events, shaped by past experience, current physical and emotional state, and perceived safety.

Interpretation is rarely neutral and rarely fully conscious.

Key question: What has this person concluded about what is happening?

Memory

The emotional archive that contributes to interpretation.

Past experiences, particularly those involving threat, loss, or dysregulation, continue to shape how present situations are understood.

Understanding

The working conclusion the person reaches about what is happening, why it is happening, and what it means for them.

Understanding does not require accuracy. It requires only that a conclusion has been formed.

Key question: What does this person believe is happening right now?

Emotion

The body's response to the understanding that has formed.

Emotion is not dysfunction. It is the nervous system preparing to respond to what it believes is occurring.

Key question: What emotional state has been activated, and what is it preparing this person to do?

Expectation

The anticipation of what is coming next, formed from everything that has moved through the chain so far.

Expectation shapes behaviour before the anticipated event has occurred.

Key question: What does this person expect to happen next?

Behaviour

The visible end of the chain.

The action, response, or change in presentation that becomes observable to others.

Key question: What need is this behaviour meeting, and how else might that need be addressed?

Static and Dynamic Links

Static links are fixed or deeply established aspects of a person's life.

Examples: age, gender, history of trauma, childhood experiences, family dynamics.

Dynamic links are influences that shift depending on situation, environment, or current state.

Examples: environment, illness, medication, substance use, external supports, insight, capacity to make decisions.

When multiple dynamic links are active simultaneously, pressure within the chain can increase rapidly.

Early Warning Signals

Behaviour rarely arrives without earlier signals. Learn to recognise:

Physical

Changes in posture, muscle tension, breathing, skin colour, stillness, or increased movement.

Communicative

Changes in tone, pace, volume, or word choice. Shorter responses. Answers that do not match the question.

Relational

Withdrawal from eye contact or engagement. Increased testing of limits. Changes in the quality of connection.

Environmental

Increased sensitivity to sensory input. Disruption to routine. Change in the person's use of or orientation to the space.

1. Regulate yourself first.

A dysregulated worker cannot co-regulate a dysregulated person. Settle your own chain before attempting to settle theirs.

2. Meet the emotion before addressing the behaviour.

Acknowledgement before correction. Attunement before expectation. Connection before redirection.

3. Reduce demand without abandoning expectation.

Temporarily reduce pressure to allow the chain to settle. Return to expectations once regulation is restored.

4. Use the environment deliberately.

Adjust what can be adjusted, whether noise, space, sensory input, or the number of people present. The environment is the first link. It can be a resource.

5. Know when to step back.

Continued engagement from a particular worker is not always helpful. Stepping back, done well, can itself be de-escalating.

6. Return after difficulty.

When the chain has settled, reconnect. A brief, genuine acknowledgement that something hard happened, without dwelling, reaffirms the relationship and lays the groundwork for change.

The Worker's Own Chain

Before each interaction, consider:

What am I bringing through the door today?

Is my own chain settled enough to be genuinely present?

What from my own history might influence how I read this situation?

What do I need to set aside in order to be available to this person?

After a difficult interaction, consider:

What was happening in my own chain during that moment?

Where did my response come from?

What would I do differently, and what support do I need to make that possible?

Team Consistency Checklist

A consistent team creates an environment in which the person being supported can develop reliable expectations.

Does the team share a common understanding of this person's chain?

Are early warning signals documented and communicated across workers?

Are responses to particular behaviours consistent across the roster?

Are disagreements about approach surfaced and discussed, or do they operate beneath the surface?

Is supervision available and genuinely supportive of workers' chains?

Is the capacity for de-escalation distributed across the team, or concentrated in one or two individuals?

A Note on Language

The Behaviour Chain Principle asks us to shift the questions we ask about behaviour.

From: Why is this person behaving like this?

To: What links in the chain have led to this moment?

From: What is wrong with this person?

To: What has this person concluded, and what has shaped that conclusion?

From: How do we stop this behaviour?

To: What need is this behaviour meeting, and how else might that need be addressed?

From: Who is to blame for this outcome?

To: What in the system contributed to this, and what can be changed?

Language shapes culture.

Culture shapes chains.

The questions we ask, consistently and over time, determine the kind of understanding that becomes possible.

Every time a worker pauses before reacting, looks earlier instead of only at what is visible, and responds to what the chain is carrying rather than what the behaviour is showing, something shifts.

Validation is not softness. Recognition is not weakness. They are the most precise tools available for repairing the links that have been under strain the longest.

The person in front of you is not their behaviour.

They are everything that led to it.

And when you can see that, everything about how you respond begins to change.

Because behaviour is never a diagnosis.

It is always a symptom.

And symptoms have a source.

Now you know where to look.

www.ingramcontent.com/pod-product-compliance
Lightning Source LLC
Chambersburg PA
CBHW061336250726
48657CB00004B/1193